VOLUME FIFTY NINE

# ADVANCES IN CHEMICAL ENGINEERING

## Process Intensification in the Manufacturing of Biotherapeutics

# ADVANCES IN CHEMICAL ENGINEERING

*Serial Editor*

**DAVIDE MOSCATELLI**
*Department of Chemistry,*
*Materials and Chemical Engineering "Giulio Natta"*
*Politecnico di Milano, Milano, Italy*

VOLUME FIFTY NINE

# ADVANCES IN CHEMICAL ENGINEERING

## Process Intensification in the Manufacturing of Biotherapeutics

Edited by

**DAVIDE MOSCATELLI**
*Department of Chemistry,*
*Materials and Chemical Engineering "Giulio Natta"*
*Politecnico di Milano, Milano, Italy*

**MATTIA SPONCHIONI**
*Department of Chemistry,*
*Materials and Chemical Engineering "Giulio Natta,"*
*Politecnico di Milano, Milano, Italy*

ELSEVIER

ACADEMIC PRESS
An imprint of Elsevier

Academic Press is an imprint of Elsevier
50 Hampshire Street, 5th Floor, Cambridge, MA 02139, United States
525 B Street, Suite 1650, San Diego, CA 92101, United States
The Boulevard, Langford Lane, Kidlington, Oxford OX5 1GB, United Kingdom
125 London Wall, London, EC2Y 5AS, United Kingdom

First edition 2022



ISBN: 978-0-323-91355-3
ISSN: 0065-2377

For information on all Academic Press publications
visit our website at https://www.elsevier.com/books-and-journals

*Publisher:* Zoe Kruze
*Acquisitions Editor:* Mariana L. Kuhl
*Developmental Editor:* Federico Paulo S. Mendoza
*Production Project Manager:* Vijayaraj Purushothaman
*Cover Designer:* Greg Harris

Typeset by STRAIVE, India

# Contents

# Contributors

**Niklas Andersson**
Department of Chemical Engineering, Lund University, Lund, Sweden

**Martina Catani**
Department of Chemical, Pharmaceutical and Agricultural Sciences, University of Ferrara, Ferrara, Italy

**Silvia Cieri**
F. Hoffmann-La Roche AG, Dept. Global Manufacturing Science and Technology, Basel, Switzerland

**Chiara De Luca**
Department of Chemical, Pharmaceutical and Agricultural Sciences, University of Ferrara, Ferrara, Italy

**Hector Marcelo Fernandez Lahore**
Jacobs University Bremen, Bremen, Germany; Luxembourg Institute of Science and Technology, Belvaux, Luxembourg

**Ismaele Fioretti**
Department of Chemistry, Materials and Chemical Engineering "Giulio Natta," Politecnico di Milano, Milano, Italy

**Joaquín Gomis Fons**
Department of Chemical Engineering, Lund University, Lund, Sweden

**Lisa-Marie Herlevi**
Jacobs University Bremen, Bremen, Germany

**Tae Keun Kim**
Department of Chemistry, Materials and Chemical Engineering "Giulio Natta," Politecnico di Milano, Milano, Italy

**João Medeiros Garcia Alcântara**
Department of Chemistry, Materials and Chemical Engineering "Giulio Natta," Politecnico di Milano, Milano, Italy

**Bernt Nilsson**
Department of Chemical Engineering, Lund University, Lund, Sweden

**Mattia Sponchioni**
Department of Chemistry, Materials and Chemical Engineering "Giulio Natta," Politecnico di Milano, Milano, Italy

# Preface

Biotherapeutics, i.e., medicinal products produced by living organisms and intended either for the treatment of diseases or for their prevention and diagnosis, are rapidly growing in importance as testified by the number of approvals and market shares. The number of yearly approved biopharmaceuticals has grown by more than a factor of 10 since the 1990s, and in 2020 the global sales reached €1.2 trillion, with a growth rate of 42% within the last decade. These figures highlight how biopharmaceuticals are on a much faster growth track compared to traditional small molecules, as it has been further demonstrated during the recent outbreak of the COVID-19 pandemic, for which 53% of the major studied therapies are indeed biologics. Among this broad family of large molecules, insulin and monoclonal antibodies are the most established representatives, but a major role is also played by mRNAs, which are considered the most promising emerging biopharmaceuticals worldwide, with the potential to lead to a concrete revolution in therapies.

Regardless of the nature of biopharmaceuticals, a common aspect is represented by the high technical complexity associated with their manufacturing, coupled with the time and resources underlying their development. These aspects lead to extremely high manufacturing costs limiting the availability of these often live-saving molecules among the population. These limitations are currently pushing toward process intensification, incentivized by the same regulatory agencies deputed to approve and allow the distribution of new biopharmaceuticals. The main output of this effort is the quality-by-design initiative, which is motivating the biopharmaceutical industry to highlight the connections between the manufacturing unit operations and the characteristics of the product. This, in turn, is stimulating a redesign of the traditional processes with advancements in many areas, from upstream to downstream processing. This revolution, also referred to as bioprocess intensification, finds its greater expression in the design of continuous unit operations and in their integration, to realize an end-to-end manufacturing process capable of improving the throughput, compress the volumes, automatize the procedures, and ensure consistent product quality attributes.

Volume 59 of the *Advances in Chemical Engineering* book series, entitled *Process Intensification in the Manufacturing of Biotherapeutics*, aims to describe the latest advances in this revolutionary trend from a process point of view, with the ultimate goal of providing the breadth of this movement that perfectly aligns with the principles of Industry 4.0. More specifically, in Chapter 1, the evolution in the design of bioreactors for the upstream processing of biopharmaceuticals is analyzed. This evolution finds its apex in perfusion bioreactors, which, combining high cell densities and continuity of the harvest recovery, is the most ideal candidate for achieving process integration. Chapters 2 and 3 then focus on the downstream processing, in particular on the effort in converting traditional single-column chromatographic purifications of biopharmaceuticals, which are limited by poor throughput, high resin cost, and low yield into a continuous process through the implementation of multicolumn countercurrent operations. While Chapter 2 encompasses the challenges and processes currently proposed for flow-through operations, Chapter 3 reports the promises of multicolumn countercurrent solvent gradient purification (MCSGP) for the polishing of biopharmaceuticals. However, chromatography is not the only unit operation to be involved in bioprocess integration. As a matter of fact, Chapter 4 reports the advances in fluidized beaded technologies for the continuous recovery and purification of biopharmaceuticals. The effort in process integration with the aim of achieving an automated and modular end-to-end manufacturing is then discussed in Chapter 5, proposing a general platform for integrated and continuous bioprocesses. Finally, Chapter 6 aims to complete a 360-degree view of the biopharma revolution with a critical analysis of the emerging trends in drug product manufacturing. In particular, the current technologies and regulations for fill–finish operations are discussed together with the macrotrends in the field, specifically related to digitalization and miniaturization.

Overall, this volume provides an in-depth analysis of the common direction undertaken by both academia and industry toward continuous and integrated operations for the manufacturing of biopharmaceuticals, expected to lead to superior performances in terms of not only productivity but also product quality, which translates into safety and efficacy for the patient.

Davide Moscatelli
Mattia Sponchioni

CHAPTER ONE

# Evolution and design of continuous bioreactors for the production of biological products

**João Medeiros Garcia Alcântara and Mattia Sponchioni***
Department of Chemistry, Materials and Chemical Engineering "Giulio Natta," Politecnico di Milano, Milano, Italy
*Corresponding author: e-mail address: mattia.sponchioni@polimi.it

## Contents



## Abstract

The bioprocessing industry is undergoing a crucial change from batch to continuous processes, backed by possible cost reductions and advantages in terms of stable product quality. Initially in this chapter, the concepts related to the birth of biotechnology are brought forward as well as some considerations related to selection of a suitable cell line depending on product type. Then, the three basic process modes for stirred tank bioreactors (i.e., batch, fed-batch and chemostat/CSTR) are exposed, including the mathematical expressions which can be used to model these processes. Perfusion-based continuous bioreactors are introduced as a way for achieving higher cell densities and therefore increasing productivities. Strategies for the development of these processes are explained, including the use of scale-down models. Finally, two case studies are brought forward. Firstly, the extracellular production of monoclonal antibodies, a rapidly expanding class of biopharmaceuticals. Secondly, the production of intracellular products via perfusion is exemplified with the case of bioplastics, specifically polyhydroxyalkanoates, one of the most researched biodegradable biopolymer.

*Advances in Chemical Engineering*, Volume 59
ISSN 0065-2377
https://doi.org/10.1016/bs.ache.2022.03.001

## 1. Introduction

The use of living organisms to produce value-added goods has a wide and ancient history. Originally exploited for the production of basic human commodities, such as bread, cheese, wine and beer, the technology has evolved toward the synthesis of complex pharmaceuticals and biological products.

The basis of the production of these more advanced categories of bioproducts is based on the development of recombinant technology. This technology was developed in the 1970s by Paul Berg, Herbest Boyer and Stanley Cohen. Central to this technology is the process of gene cloning, which coupled with the fast development of DNA sequencing techniques allowed the genetic modification of naturally occurring microorganisms to produce any product of interest. Specifically, DNA sequencing allowed for the study of the structures and regulation of individual genes, giving birth to modern biotechnology.

In the following years, another very import technique for gene manipulation was discovered: Polymerase Chain Reaction (PCR). This technique is very much used until today, for a variety of objectives, including diagnostics. PCR based-detection of SARS-Cov-2 is still very much the gold standard. However, its importance in biotechnology should not be underrated, given the important advances this technique enabled in the accomplishment of gene cloning with ease.

Coupling these two important discoveries, it is possible to genetically engineer a host microorganism to produce the bioproduct desired. Specifically, the DNA sequence that codes for the product of interest is inserted into a cell line that is then able to translate that sequence and produce the product, through the already existing machinery inside the cell. The introduction of this exogenous DNA sequence is done through the process of transfection. The specific technology employed depends slightly on the type of cell (bacterial, yeast, plant or animal), for the specific case of animal cells it can be done via: direct transfer by physical transfection, chemical transfection, transduction, or by packing the DNA inside a bacterium (Brown, 2010).

Having the knowledge to genetically engineer a cell line, the question of how to select that production cell line is posed. Initially, this strain should satisfy certain basic requirements: not be a pathogen, clear genomic background, be easy of genetical manipulation, not produce toxins, have a fast growth, and, ideally, have a wide substrate utilization.

Most bioproducts are produced either via a bacterial or a mammalian cell line. Specifically, the choice of which will mostly depend on the product. If the product is simple (e.g., a small molecule), normally, a bacterial cell line would be selected. This is justified by their faster growth and cheaper media, which then results in higher productivity and lower costs. However, if instead the product is complex, such as therapeutic proteins, a mammalian cell line is selected. Even though, their cultivation is more complex, presents lower productivities and higher costs, there are certain factors which make mammalian cells a better choice. Specifically, for the production of proteins, even though the exact same sequence of amino acids could be achieved in a bacterial cell line, bacteria do not have the required machinery to introduce the posttranslational modifications which occur in mammalian cells. These modifications have then an effect on the immune response and action of therapeutic product and therefore justify the higher cost.

In order to produce bioproducts effectively, ad hoc equipment was developed. Even though mammalian cell lines grow naturally in adherent conditions (e.g., on petri dishes), commercial cell lines have been adapted to grow in suspension cultures, which allows for higher cell densities, since the maximum density achievable in a bioreactor is not limited by its surface, as the whole volume can be exploited in this case. On the other hand, bacterial cell lines can naturally grow in suspension. Therefore, in the following chapter the focus will be put on the use of stirred tank bioreactors for the production of bioproducts.

## 2. From batch to continuous

### 2.1 Basic bioreactor concepts

In order to take advantage of the possibilities unveiled by recombinant technology, ever more efficient productive process units were developed: bioreactors.

Bioreactors are the process units in which the product of interest is formed, encompassing a wide array of scales (across development stages and industries) and in applications. The stirred tank reactor is the most used type in industrial processes and will be the type discussed in this work. This type of bioreactor is characterized by having a central mechanical stirrer (with different types of turbines, depending on the application) which is responsible for mixing and contributes to aeration. Normally, these bioreactors are coupled with a variety of sensors which allow the maintenance of stable process conditions through simple control strategies. Normally, these include at least temperature, pH and dissolved oxygen (DO) (in the case the culture is aerobic) sensors. However, even more advanced sensors can be added which can monitor continuously cell density using capacitance probes (Teixeira et al., 2009). Furthermore, in the last years, there has been a high increase in the interest of introducing spectrometer probes (such as NIR, IR or Raman) into bioreactors, which through multivariate modeling can generate online data on cell density and metabolite concentrations (Abu-Absi et al., 2011; Gouveia et al., 2017).

Over the years, different bioreactor operating modes have been developed, normally defined by the way fresh media is fed into the reactor. Hence, three major groups can be distinguished: batch, fed-batch and continuous (Doran, 1995). The batch operation is the simplest one for conducting a fermentation, not only in terms of equipment but also in terms of process management. It is characterized by the addition of the culture media with all necessary nutrients to sustain the production as well as of the inoculum at the start and removal of all products at the end of the reaction. Since the nutrients are loaded at the beginning of the process, they limit the maximum extent of the culture, as well as the maximum achievable productivity. This is even more limiting considering that the amount of nutrients loaded in the bioreactor cannot be indefinitely increased, but is limited to an upper threshold to achieve favorable cell growth conditions. This motivated the sustained feeding of fresh media throughout the whole process, in a fed-batch operation. This process allowed to increase the cell density inside the bioreactor, and consequently the productivity compared to the batch operation. Despite the advantages, it is still limited by the drawbacks of a discontinuous process, such as batch-to-batch variability of the product, which is even more severe for bioprocesses given the strict dependency of the produced molecule from the media composition, necessity of interrupting the production for recovering the product, dead times associated with reactor cleaning and charging of cells and media. In addition, peculiar to this kind of operations is the accumulation of metabolites throughout the process, which can have a negative impact on cell proliferation and growth. To overcome these limitations, continuous stirred tank bioreactors were introduced. In continuous processes, fresh media (containing all the necessary nutrients) is continuously fed into the bioreactor and culture media is pumped out at the same flow rate, in order to maintain the bioreactor volume constant. This suppresses the variability and quality fluctuations typical of discontinuous operations, ensuring a harvest with reliable quality, important for the downstream processing it will undergo to (Warikoo et al., 2012). The cost to be paid for such advancement is an improved process complexity, which should be carefully considered.

A detailed description of the three main process configurations is provided in the following sections.

## 2.2 Batch bioreactors

Batch bioreactors are the simplest form of fermentation. Consisting of a closed tank with constant volume, this bioreactor has no inlet or outlet streams (see Fig. 1A). A cellular inoculum is inserted into the tank containing fresh media and the product is harvested when the titer has reached a maximum. The fresh media that was inserted in the beginning must contain all the nutrients (i.e., carbon, nitrogen source, salts, growth factor, trace elements, among others) to support the cell growth during the lifespan of the process. As in other bioreactors, process parameters such as pH, dissolved oxygen, temperature and stirring are online controlled. In most cases, the culture reaches a maximum of cell density (and hence titer) when one or more nutrients are exhausted, impeding further cell growth.

Specifically, a typical batch culture undergoes four distinct stages: lag, exponential (or log), stationary and death. The lag phase consists of an adaptation of the cellular mass to different culture conditions. The lag phase is followed by the exponential stage, in which the cell density increases exponentially with time. The stationary phase follows, in which the cell density is

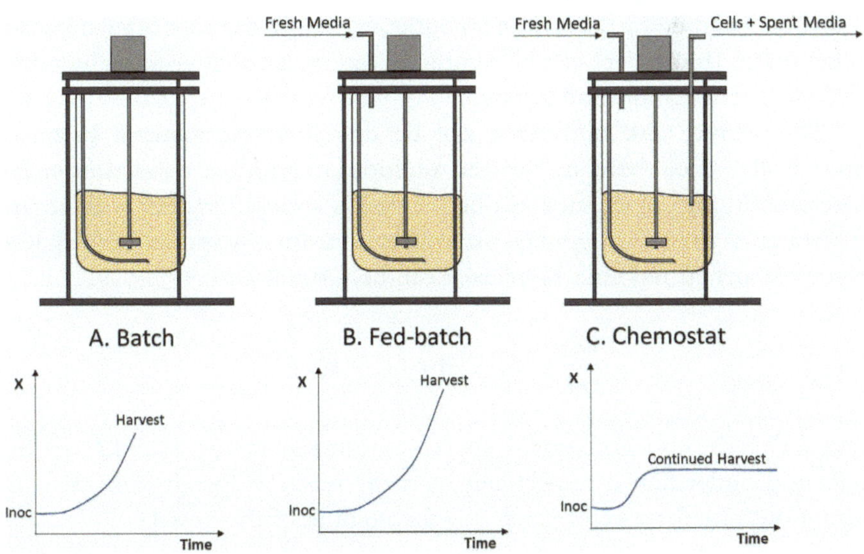


**Fig. 1** Schematic representation of the inlet and outlet streams and temporal behavior of cell density of the different process strategies for the operation of stirred tank bioreactors. A: Batch, B: Fed-Batch, C: Chemostat or CSTR.

constant and the growth and death rate are in equilibrium. Normally, a batch reaction is terminated (product is harvested) at the transition between the exponential and the stationary phase, where a maximum of cell density and product concentration is reached. This is done in order to increase the bioreactor utilization. However, if not terminated prematurely, the cell culture will also undergo the death stage, in which there is a decrease of cell density due to lack of nutrients and accumulation of toxic metabolites (Doran, 1995).

The lag phase can be shortened via the inoculum preparation process. Specifically, a cell line is normally stored via cryopreservation in small samples. In order to produce a suitable cell mass for inoculation to the bioreactor, the original cryopreserved cells undergo a process called expansion. Here, the cells are cultured in fresh media, and as cell numbers increase, also the volume of the culture recipient increases. If in the last culture steps the expansion media is closely related to the formulation of the media used in the production bioreactor and the culture conditions are similar, the lag phase will be shorter since the cells have already been adapted to the new extracellular environment. The decrease in lag phase will then increase productivity, given that it increases the bioreactor utilization rate (Hu, 2012a).

This accumulation of toxic metabolites can already affect the culture even before, causing a premature end of the exponential phase. The accumulation is caused by the lack of an outlet stream. In the case of mammalian cell culture, this impact can be significant and is normally caused by accumulation of ammonia and lactate.

This stirred tank bioreactor can be described via material balances. Specifically, since there are no feed additions or product extraction in the batch mode, this bioreactor can be viewed as a closed system with regard to the liquid phase. The general material balance for any species in the liquid phase for any stirred tank bioreactor can be written as:

$$\frac{dC_i}{dt} = F_i \cdot C_i + r_i \cdot V - F_o \cdot C_o$$

where $C_i$ is the concentration of species $i$ in the bioreactor, $F_i$ and $F_o$ are the inlet and outlet flows, respectively, $r_i$ is the reaction (production or consumption) rate for species $i$ and $V$ is the volume of the vessel.

The stirred tank bioreactor, operating in batch mode, can therefore be described by a simple ordinary differential equation (ODE) system, without any entrance or exit:

$$\frac{dX_v}{dt} = \mu \cdot X_v - k_d X_v$$

$$\frac{dX_d}{dt} = k_d \cdot X_v$$

$$\frac{dS}{dt} = -k_S \cdot X_v$$

$$\frac{dP}{dt} = k_P \cdot X_v$$

where $X_v$ and $X_d$ are the viable and dead cell density, respectively, $S$ is the main carbon source concentration and $P$ is the product concentration. With regard to mass balance for the viable cell density, both growth and death rates coefficients are considered, $\mu$ and $k_d$, respectively. Finally, $k$ represents the reaction rate coefficient for the other species.

## 2.3 Fed-batch bioreactors

This type of bioreactors is an improvement with respect to batch. This is implemented by the addition of an inlet stream which feeds concentrated fresh media containing essential nutrients throughout the process (see Fig. 1B). An action of this type can reduce the likelihood of substrate limitation and hence lead to an increase in the lifespan of the culture. Other cases, in which this type of bioreactor is beneficial include: cultures in which the additions of potentially toxic nutrients is needed, therefore keeping them below toxic concentration levels; in the case of nongrowth associated products, in which the objective is to prolong the stationary phase of the culture, or even the supply of a different media in order to maximize product formation; when very high cell densities are warranted and therefore would be unviable to supply all the carbon source needed at the start of the culture since it would lead to inhibitory concentrations.

As in the previous case, the product is harvested when the titer has reached a maximum.

Several feeding policies can be implemented, either continuous or discontinuous, depending on the nutritional needs of the culture. Normally, feeds are added as concentrated solutions, in order to avoid the dilution of the culture.

Also, this type of bioreactor does not possess an outlet stream, therefore it also incurs into the issue of culture inhibition due to toxic metabolite accumulation.

In the same way as for the batch bioreactor and with the same meaning of the different parameters, this system can also be described by a combination of the mass balances for viable and dead cell density, substrate (carbon source) and product concentrations. However, in this case there is an addition of fresh media into the bioreactor, leading to the addition of the respective term in the mass balance with regard to the substrate and an extra equation describing the increase in the volume of the bioreactor:

$$\frac{dX_v \cdot V}{dt} = \mu \cdot X_v \cdot V - k_d X_v \cdot V$$

$$\frac{dX_d \cdot V}{dt} = k_d \cdot X_v \cdot V$$

$$\frac{dS \cdot V}{dt} = -k_S \cdot X_v \cdot V + F_i \cdot S_i$$

$$\frac{dP \cdot V}{dt} = k_P \cdot X_v \cdot V$$

$$\frac{dV}{dt} = F_i$$

## 2.4 CSTR

The most common implementation of a continuous bioreactor is the CSTR or chemostat. An inlet stream supplies fresh media which contains all the necessary nutrients, and an outlet stream removes products, cells and spent media from the bioreactor at the same flow rate as the inlet stream in order to keep the volume constant (see Fig. 1C). At the start, upon inoculation, the bioreactor undergoes a startup phase in which the cell density increases until reaching a steady state. In steady state conditions the concentrations of viable and dead cells, substrates, and products are constant in time indefinitely. Hence the name of chemostat. However, it is normally infeasible to keep a chemostat running for more than a couple of weeks since perturbations can occur. This is either due to mechanical failures or even caused by random mutations of the microorganisms, which leads to the occurrence of subcultures which can change the behavior of the bioreactor.

One of the most important parameters in CSTR is the dilution rate, which corresponds to the inverse of the media residence time in the reactor:

$$D = F_i/V$$

In similarity to the other operating modes of stirred tank bioreactor, also the CSTR can be described via a system of ODEs. In this case, an inlet and outlet term need to be considered, hence, assuming that the inlet stream is sterile:

$$\frac{dX_v \cdot V}{dt} = \mu \cdot X_v \cdot V - k_d X_v \cdot V - F_o X_v$$

$$\frac{dX_d \cdot V}{dt} = k_d \cdot X_v \cdot V - F_o X_d$$

$$\frac{dS \cdot V}{dt} = -k_S \cdot X_v \cdot V + F_i \cdot S_i - F_o S$$

$$\frac{dP \cdot V}{dt} = k_P \cdot X_v \cdot V - F_o P$$

$$\frac{dV}{dt} = F_i - F_o$$

Being $F_i$ and $F_o$ the volumetric inlet and outlet flow rates, respectively. Assuming a death rate much lower than the dilution rate, it is possible to conclude that $\mu \cong D$. This leads to the definition of the maximum dilution rate, above which the cell density starts to drop. This maximum dilution rate defines the so-called wash-out conditions. In practical terms, the dilution rate cannot go above the cellular growth rate (or above a safety margin of the former) in order to avoid depletion of the cells inside the reactor, and then a drop in the productivity. This limitation generated the motivation for the creation of high cell density bioreactors, where perfusion bioreactors are included.

## 2.5 Perfusion cultures

Inserted in a current, however nonunanimous (Croughan et al., 2015; Karst et al., 2018; Konstantinov and Cooney, 2015), change from batch to continuous manufacturing, perfusion bioreactors present a suitable system to culture mammalian cells, in order to produce high value pharmaceuticals. As mentioned previously, in a general continuous culture, the so-called chemostat, fresh media is continuously added, while culture liquid containing nutrients, metabolites and cells are seamlessly removed at the same rate, in order to keep the reactor volume constant. The main limitation of this reactor system is the maximum dilution rate at which it can operate. If this parameter is higher than the cellular growth rate, then the cells will wash-out and the production of the molecule of interest will be compromised. Perfusion bioreactors, in turn, allow the operation at higher dilution rates by making use of a cell retention/recycling device that permits that the cells remain in the bioreactor, increasing throughput through superior cell densities. Another advantage is that, in comparable dilution rates, perfusion is a much more stable operating mode than the chemostat (Konstantinov et al., 1996). Thus, perfusion technology enables the continuous addition of fresh media and the continuous removal of the product and by-products, and thus allows the achievement of higher viable cell densities and increased volumetric productivities even when compared to the fed-batch technology (Bonham-Carter and Shevitz, 2011; Hu, 2012b; Karst et al., 2016).

In a general perfusion culture, there is one input, the feed, and two outputs: the bleed and the harvest (Fig. 2). The feed allows the continued supply of fresh media to the bioreactor and the harvest, located after the cell retention device, permits the uninterrupted evacuation of spent media, which eventually contains the product whenever it is secreted extracellularly, as well as any toxic metabolites that could limit cell proliferation. On the other hand, the bleed has the function of removing cell-containing culture broth directly from the reactor, enabling the control of the cellular density in the bioreactor and to collect eventual intracellular products. Hence, operating at a constant cell density, after achieving steady-state conditions, the cellular growth rate and the bleed rate will be the same (Hu, 2012b).

The most important process parameters in perfusion are the perfusion rate (*P*) and the viable cell density (VCD or $X_v$). The perfusion rate is defined

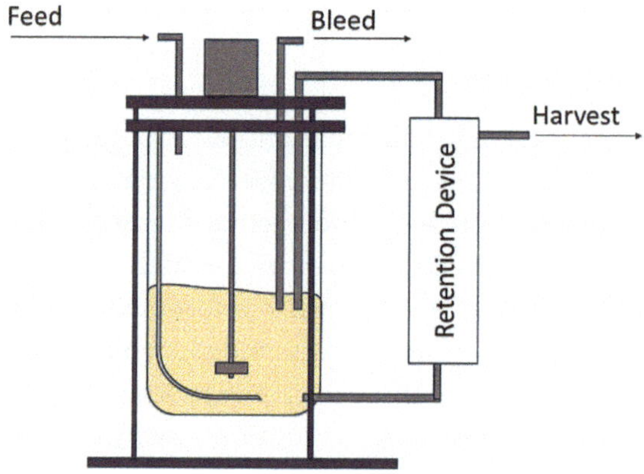


**Fig. 2** Schematic representation of the inlet and outlet streams of a perfusion bioreactor. The feed inlet stream allows for the addition of fresh media, the harvest is a cell-free outlet stream from where extracellular product is extracted and the bleed is a cell-containing outlet stream used to maintain cell-density at the set point.

as the flow of fresh media entering the bioreactor ($P=F_i$). Taking this definition into consideration the mass balances for this type of bioreactor are very similar to the case of the CSTR, with the difference that two outlet flow rates exist, bleed ($B$) and harvest ($H$):

$$\frac{dX_v \cdot V}{dt} = \mu \cdot X_v \cdot V - k_d \cdot X_v \cdot V - B \cdot X_v$$

$$\frac{dX_d \cdot V}{dt} = k_d \cdot X_v \cdot V - B \cdot X_d$$

$$\frac{dS \cdot V}{dt} = -k_S \cdot X_v \cdot V + P \cdot S_i - H \cdot S - B \cdot S$$

$$\frac{dP \cdot V}{dt} = k_P \cdot X_v \cdot V - H \cdot P - B \cdot P$$

$$\frac{dV}{dt} = F_i - B - H$$

Furthermore, the concept of cell-specific perfusion rate (CSPR) can be defined, which expresses the flow of media experienced by a single cell, and hence defined as:

$$CSPR = \frac{P}{X_v}$$

Since one of the major cost drivers in perfusion cultures is the media, normally this process is translated into having the lowest possible CSPR. This minimization procedure is of course limited by the minimum amount of nutrients required by the cell to grow, proliferate and produce the product of interest. Therefore, a minimum CSTR at which the perfusion process can be conducted is typically defined as $CSPR_{min}$. This is a function of the media composition, and hence an effort has been done in order to reduce as much as possible this value, in order to save nutrient costs.

The choice of the cell retention device depends on several factors, including the way cells grow (if in single-cell suspension, or if in aggregates), the required harvest rate and the scale of the operation. Different devices have been developed over the years, which perform retention based on different cellular physical or chemical characteristics, for example: size, density, electrical charges, dielectric constant and surface properties. Size-based separations are those ensuring the highest cell retention and are mostly based on the concept of filtration. These devices include cross-flow filters, hollow fibers (both Tangential Flow Filtration (TFF) and Alternating Tangential Flow (ATF), see Fig. 3), controlled shear filtration, vortex-flow filtration

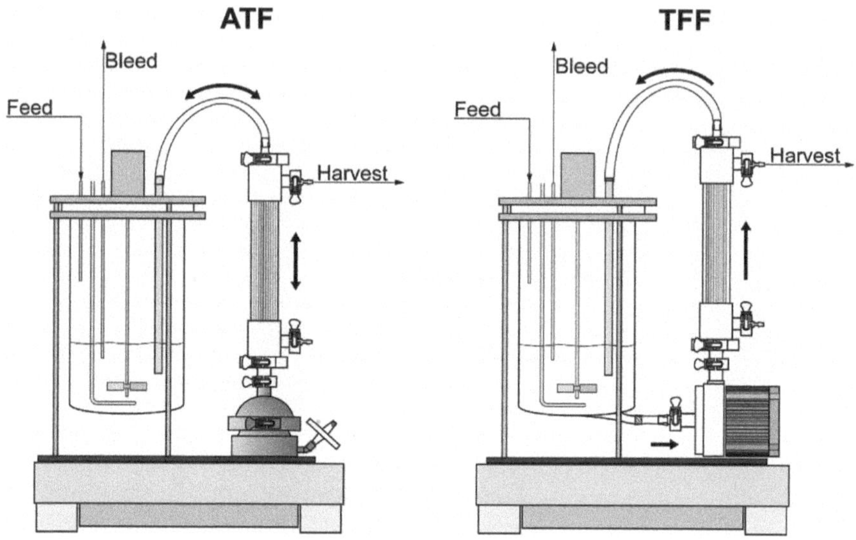


**Fig. 3** Schematic representation of perfusion bioreactors which use as retention device a hollow fiber as filtration method, differing on which pump is used: alternating tangential flow filtration (ATF) uses a diaphragm pump and tangential flow filtration (TFF) uses a centrifugal pump. *Reproduced with permission from Karst DJ, Serra E, Villiger TK, Soos M, Morbidelli M: Characterization comparison of ATF and TFF in stirred bioreactors for continuous mammalian cell culture processes,* Biochem Eng J *110:17–26, 2016. Copyright Elsevier 2016.*

and spin-filters. Retention based on density include gravity settlers, centrifuges, enhanced settling by acoustic waves and hydrocyclones. Other methods exist, but the ones mentioned include the most used (Castilho and Medronho, 2002; Hu, 2012b; Voisard et al., 2003; Woodside et al., 1998).

It should be pointed out that not all these processes offer a complete retention of the cells. According to Voisard et al. (Voisard et al., 2003), in a scale until 250 L, the most adequate cell retention device are the ones that make use of hollow-fiber modules. In this group there are two alternative technologies: TFF and ATF. The main difference between the two is that in a TFF setting the flow through the hollow fiber is unidirectional. The device is inserted in an external loop, through which the broth is recirculated through a centrifugal pump whose maximum rate is governed by the mechanical stress the cells can tolerate. With this configuration, a recurrent problem is the fouling of the membrane. This can be alleviated with the ATF device, applying an alternate flow at the membrane through alternatively positive and negative pressure cycles implemented through a diaphragm pump (see Fig. 3). It is believed that this alternated flow characteristic of the ATF decreases the fouling of the membrane (Clincke et al., 2013; Hu, 2012b; Karst et al., 2016; Voisard et al., 2003). Although it has been shown by Wang et al. (Wang et al., 2017) that this comparison is highly dependent on the degree of shear stress that the type of pump used in the TFF module exerts on the cells, this is open to discussion since Karst et al. (Karst et al., 2016) reported contradictory findings in similar set-ups.

Given the inherent complexity of perfusion cultures, process development is an incredibly labor intensive and complex task. This is true due to an inherently high number of experimental factors to be considered, leading to intensive experimental campaigns. This stage integrates several tasks, such as cell-line selection, perfusion specific media development and operational parameter optimization (Wolf et al., 2020).

As it might be expected if all of the experimental trials would be conducted at the process scale (or even at a pilot or bench-top/laboratory scale) the cost would be extremely high. Hence, a number of scale-down methods were developed. These try to mimic conditions at the production scale to experiments ranging from 500 mL to a few microliters, with varying levels of automatization.

In particular, scale-down models aim to reproduce the behavior of production scale bioreactors which can be in the order of tens to thousands of liters in order to save the costs associated to the expensive media and cells as well as the effort in managing such a complex system.

There are a few requirements for the small systems of choice to be good scale-down models of bioreactors. These include the easiness of working with them, low need of human intervention, low cost per unit, and high throughput. The scale-down models which fit these requirements can then range from less to more automatized ones e.g., from spin tubes to automated microbioreactors. They also range different scales: from a few microliters (deep-well plates) to some milliliters (spin tubes), and to liters (automated microbioreactors) (Bielser et al., 2019).

Starting from the smaller scale, 96 or 12 deep well plates have the potentiality to run many experiments simultaneously on only one plate. These are very useful for example for cell line selection or for media optimization, in which there are a lot of possibilities to be considered and this allows for a quick and easy way of determining which are the best possible candidates for further experimentation. Moreover, these deep well plates can be automatized and integrated into already commercially available pipetting platforms which can reduce the manual labor involved. Then, as the number of possible candidates of or conjunction of experimental factors reduces further experimentation can be performed at higher scales, e.g. spin-tubes.

Spin-tubes have already a working volume of few milliliters and are among the most used scale-down models (Wolf et al., 2018). Oxygen transfer occurs through the surface of the liquid and hence the surface area can be toggled by varying the shaking speed or the culture volume in the tube. All operations are done manually by an operator in sterile conditions in a biosafety cabinet. In order to mimic perfusion in a semicontinuous fashion, these tubes require daily operations and go through several stages (see Fig. 4). Firstly, a sample is taken to measure VCD and metabolite concentrations. Based on the defined value of VCD to be established in the model, a consequent bleed is performed. Then the spin-tubes are spun-down via the action of a centrifuge, allowing for removal of cell-free harvest. Finally, fresh media is added to maintain culture volume and the cell pellet resuspended. Several authors have confirmed the reliability of these scale-down models in relation to the current gold standard of bench-scale bioreactors (Bielser et al., 2019; Wolf et al., 2018).

Recently, automated microbioreactors (ambr) were developed with perfusion capabilities. These small bioreactors (15–500 mL) already allow for continuous flows and can extremely reliably mimic conditions at a higher scale (Janoschek et al., 2019; Jin et al., 2021). In these, oxygen transfer is no longer done via the superficial area on top of the liquid but is delivered via a sparger. Furthermore, since it is possible to place multiple sensors inside these bioreactors, other process parameters such as pH and DO can be directly controlled. These bioreactors are highly automated in sampling and feeding, requiring a very low level of operator intervention.

An important factor that needs to be experimentally optimized for perfusion cell cultures is the media composition. Initially, most media for mammalian cell culture included nutrients from natural sources, such as serum, plasma

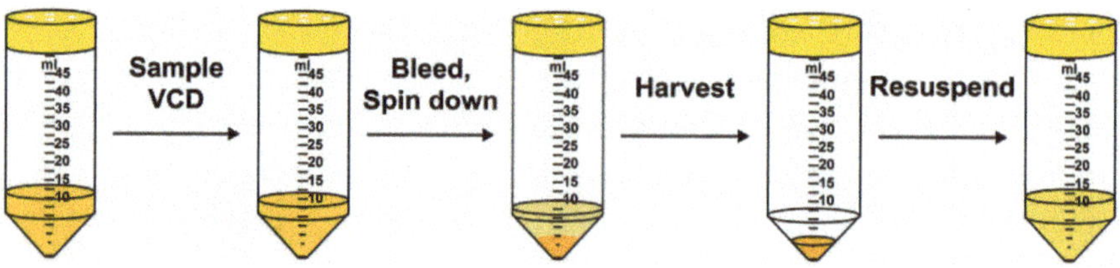


**Fig. 4** Representation of the process used to simulate a perfusion process using scale-down models, in this case, spin-tubes. *Reproduced with permission from Wolf MKF, Lorenz V, Karst DJ, Souquet J, Broly H, Morbidelli M: Development of a shake-tube-based scale-down model for perfusion cultures,* Biotechnol Bioeng, *2018. Copyright John Wiley & Sons 2018.*

or vegetable or animal extracts. However, these carried some drawbacks, as the most relevant of which is the high lot-to-lot variation leading to significant differences in culture outcomes. Given this, the industry has ever more switched to chemically-defined media, where composition can be much better controlled with exact concentrations of all the necessary nutrients: vitamins, growth factors, carbon source, and nitrogen source.

Media compositions defined for previously existing fed-batch processes can be used as an initial starting point for perfusion media development. However, due to the different process objectives, some changes are seldom needed. In order to facilitate media development, the concept of media depth was developed. This relates to one of the most important parameters in perfusion cultures: the CSPR. This parameter signifies the minimum quantity of media needed to support a given VCD. Hence, the objective should be to develop a media which shows a maximum media depth. Normally this is done in conjunction with CSPR optimization.

$$\text{Medium depth} = \frac{1}{CSPR_{min}}$$

There are two ways of reducing the CSPR: either by lowering the perfusion rate or by increasing the VCD (see Fig. 5). The former is called the "push-to-low" approach and involves step-wise reductions in the amount of media fed, the media composition can also be changed from iteration to iteration,

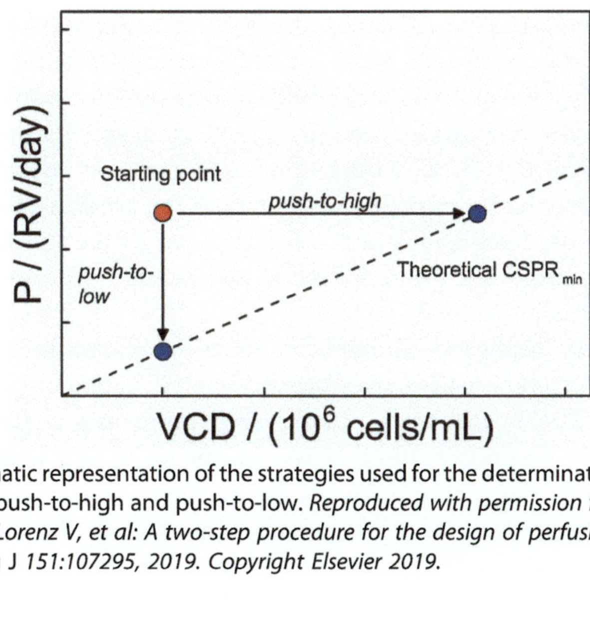


**Fig. 5** Schematic representation of the strategies used for the determination of the minimum CSPR, push-to-high and push-to-low. *Reproduced with permission from Wolf MKF, Pechlaner A, Lorenz V, et al: A two-step procedure for the design of perfusion bioreactors,* Biochem Eng J *151:107295, 2019. Copyright Elsevier 2019.*

by decreasing the ratio of basal to enriched media (Konstantinov et al., 2006). The use of more enriched media allows the same volume of media to support more cells (increased "media depth"). The latter approach, "push-to-high," makes use of an enriched media to increase the VCD at a constant perfusion rate, also in a step-wise manner (Xu et al., 2017). These approaches can even be combined in order to determine the best operating conditions for the perfusion bioreactor (Wolf et al., 2018). With regard to the first approach mentioned, if the CSPR is reduced then residence time of the product in the reactor will be higher, hence the lability (a possible measure is the half-life) of the product should also be considered when optimizing the culture (Konstantinov et al., 2006). According to Konstantinov et al. (Konstantinov et al., 2006), the main points to be researched further, in order to overcome the problems that a decrease in perfusion rate carries are: (1) media that can sustain more cells per volume added, (2) evaluation of extremely low perfusion rates on the physiology and productivity of the cells and (3) the protection of the product from degradation.

In a standard continuous process, the goal of the operation is to control the process parameters in order to keep and maintain a steady-state (for the sake of correctness it should be pointed out that when referring to a steady-state, one is actually referring to a pseudo-steady-state) (Jungbauer et al., 2017). In fact, this type of cell culture system allows the continuous cultivation of mammalian cell cultures at high viable cell densities, which is beneficial for overall product yields and allows the produced product to have a homogeneous quality (Karst et al., 2017a,b; Warikoo et al., 2012). Accordingly, if a steady-state is achieved, the quality attributes of the product will have to remain in a similar range during the time of the operation. Dealing with constant quality harvest is beneficial mainly for the design and implementation of all the downstream operations that are typically in place for satisfying the market purity requirements on the produced biologic. The avoidance of the fluctuations in the composition of the stream that these units need to handle allow more stable and reliable processes as well as simplify the quality control.

Given that steady-state multiplicity exists in mammalian cell culture (Europa et al., 2000), it has been observed in CHO cultures by Karst et al. (Karst et al., 2017b) that the metabolic fingerprints in a perfusion culture are steady-state dependent. In other words, one set of operating conditions will correspond to a specific product quality profile and also specific metabolic input and output rates. This is especially important in the framework of quality-by-design (QBD), in order to link (critical) process parameters (CPPs) to the (critical) quality attributes (CQAs), also enabling higher process understanding and, eventually, facilitating the implementation of a control strategy (EMA, 2009; FDA, 2012; Karst et al., 2018). However, it should be pointed out that in a closed loop process, for the CQAs to remain in their specifications, the manipulated variables will be changed over time, instead of having steady-state values, due to natural (e.g., environmental) perturbation to the process. The manipulated variables are the degrees of freedom which are available for control purposes, for example the stirrer speed, volumetric air flow, harvest, bleed and perfusion rates, media composition, among others (Myerson et al., 2015).

Regarding control parameters, this set includes most parameters typical of a bioprocess, such as pH, temperature, DO, media composition, concentration of metabolites in solution, among others. However, in perfusion processes the CSPR also is shown to be a very important control parameter. Some groups (Dowd et al., 2003; Fernandez-de-Cossio-Diaz et al., 2017) have even reported that in order to maintain a given metabolic state the parameter to control is in fact the CSPR. Also, in terms of pH control it has been reported (Xu and Chen, 2016) that in a given range the pH is regulated by the cell metabolism and that external pH control is not required. The reactor temperature is also an important parameter, since it can have a significant effect on the cell specific productivity (Chuppa et al., 1997). Also reported has been the monitoring and control of the levels of glucose and lactate in solution, which can also work as an early indicator for contamination. In fact, the cell specific glucose uptake rate can also be used as an indicator of steady-state operation (Angepat et al., 2005; Ozturk et al., 1997).

However, some research groups have investigated nonsteady state perfusion cultures. These research groups argue that this mode implies long development and manufacturing times, extended process performance qualification (PPQ), large media consumption and concerns on the variability of the product quality and contamination (Coffman et al., 2017). In terms of the development of the control strategy the latter case can bring increased difficulties, since instead of a fixed set of set-points that need to be maintained throughout the duration of the culture, in a nonsteady-state operation the set-point inherently changes as a function of time, hence the necessity of employing a set-point tracking. However, it can become a simpler operation due to the removal of the bleeding-derived increased complexity, a process of this kind is in fact in the transition between fed-batch and steady-state perfusion.

Nonetheless, it also should be pointed out that in true end-to-end continuous manufacturing the system must be in stationary state, however an adaptive control strategy should be in place in each unit to counteract possible upstream perturbations (Jungbauer et al., 2017).

In the next sections, examples of the production of therapeutic proteins and polyhydroxyalkanoates using perfusion cell cultures will be discussed.

## 3. Production of monoclonal antibodies

Mammalian cell perfusion processes are particularly suitable for the production of extracellular products, such as secreted therapeutic proteins. A relevant example is represented by the production of monoclonal antibodies (mAbs), which are typically obtained from engineered Chinese Hamster Ovary (CHO) cells. The need for intensification in the production of mAbs is driven by a compound annual growth rate (CAGR) above 10%, with a total market size that has overcome 100 billion USD in 2019 (Diallo et al., 2020). This growing demand for mAbs was further boosted in the last years by the COVID-19 pandemic. The great effort in finding effective treatments to this disease led to repurpose over 60 mAb-based therapies originally approved and marketed for other indications and to develop new biopharmaceuticals (Kaplon and Reichert, 2021).

The development of perfusion processes is particularly suitable for ensuring high productivity and reduced fluctuations in the CQAs of the product, which, combined to the continuity of the product recovery, is convenient for the connection of upstream and downstream processing (DSP), in the realization of an integrated process (Narayanan et al., 2022). With this respect, a general scheme for a continuous bioprocessing facility for the production of monoclonal antibodies includes the perfusion bioreactor, several chromatographic separation steps, a filtration unit, optional virus inactivation units and hold tanks for the medium, the finished product and intermediates.

Perfusion processes aimed at the production of mAbs from CHO cells have been first described by Warikoo et al. in 2012 (Warikoo et al., 2012). In this seminal work, the bioreactor was provided with an ATF cell retention system and operated at a perfusion rate between 2 and 3 RV/day. With a CSPR of 40–50 pL/(cell day), the authors anticipated the huge effort spent in minimizing the nutrient provision, which would have been carried out in the following decade. Even so, the operation reached steady-state after 30 culture days and the VCD was maintained almost constant to

50 Mcells/mL for further 40 days. Despite steady-state conditions were maintained for the VCD, this was not the case for the volumetric productivity, which peaked at 1 g/(L day) after 30 days and then slowly decreased for reasons not investigated by the authors. Nonetheless, this introduces a key point for the management of continuous culture processes for long time, which is the likelihood of modifications at the level of the cell genome that could be the cause for the observed decrease in mAb productivity. Cell random mutations can introduce variability in terms of product attributes, mainly in the glycosylation pattern (Feidl et al., 2020). It is then essential to constantly monitor the harvest and design a control strategy able to predict and promptly react to such drifts.

The merit of the authors also lies in having integrated, for the first time, the perfusion bioreactor with a chromatographic capture step operated in continuous (Fig. 6A). The downstream section comprised an ultrafiltration device and a four-column periodic countercurrent (PCC) operation. To compensate the different flow rates of the upstream and downstream sections, a surge bag was placed between the two. The downstream section was operated for 30 days after the perfusion bioreactor reached steady-state and the possibility of maintaining stable recovery and the CQAs of the product leaving the process was verified by measuring the aggregation, potency, protein A leakage from the resin and host cell proteins. The authors demonstrated how these CQAs reached steady-state and how that could be preserved for the whole duration of the production campaign. In particular, high product recovery, above 90%, could be achieved, with levels of contaminants within the acceptable range for distribution.

Remarkably, the first end-to-end integrated process for the production of mAbs and based on perfusion cell culture was reported by Godawat et al. (Godawat et al., 2015). Compared to the previous example, the downstream section integrated both capture and polishing operations conducted in continuous. Between the two, a low pH hold served as virus inactivation step. With this DSP train, the drug substance could be produced with a low content in host cell proteins, whose concentration in the purification units was knocked down by 4 orders of magnitude compared to the eluent from the bioreactor. In addition, the product quality could was consistent for over 30 days, confirming the possibility of exploiting perfusion CHO cell culture processes for prolonged duration.

It is worth highlighting that the stability of the production cell line is notoriously a critical point when aiming at an integrated process. In fact, fluctuations in the productivity of the bioreactor or in the product CQAs

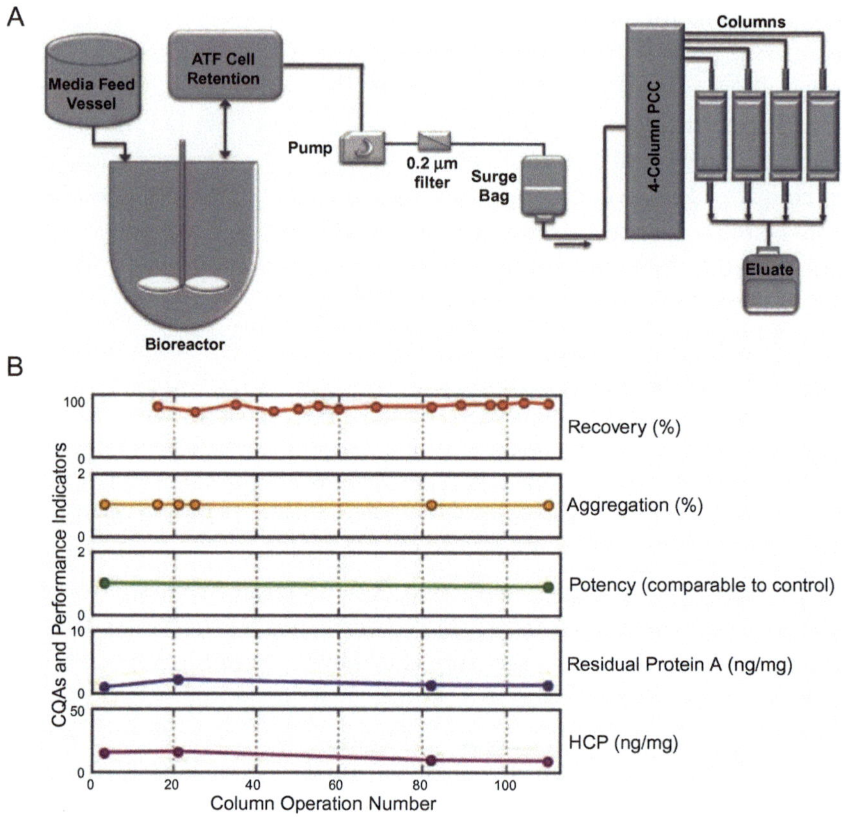


**Fig. 6** (A) Schematic representation of the continuous integrated mAb process comprising a perfusion bioreactor and a downstream section with an ultrafiltration and a four-column PCC chromatographic capture step. (B) Recovery and CQAs measured for the product leaving the process, including aggregation, potency, leaked protein A and host cell proteins. *Reproduced with permission from Warikoo V, Godawat R, Brower K, et al: Integrated continuous production of recombinant therapeutic proteins,* Biotechnol Bioeng *109(12):3018–3029, 2012. Copyright John Wiley & Sons, 2012.*

related to variability in the media or to drifts in the biological system significantly affect the optimal conduction of the downstream operations. To compensate such fluctuations, it is essential that the different units of the process communicate with each other through a system of sensors measuring the CQAs of the product and actuators that directly intervene on the specific unit set point. In a recent work, Feidl et al. (Feidl et al., 2020) developed a digital supervisory control and data acquisition (SCADA) system for the monitoring and control of an integrated process for the production of mAbs. The process comprised a perfusion bioreactor connected to a chromatographic capture step, a virus inactivation unit and two polishing steps based on ion exchange chromatography. The introduction of different online sensors and at-line high-performance liquid chromatography (HPLC) units allowed to monitor in real time the main outputs of the reactor and each purification unit and then to intervene on specific set points. In particular, at the level of the bioreactor, the VCD could be adjusted to compensate the loss in productivity associated with instability of the cell line. Moreover, fluctuations in the harvest titer served for the automatic regulation of the residence time in the following capture step. Finally, a strict control on the pH downstream to the virus inactivation unit was applied to minimize protein aggregation and to allow constant product CQAs to the polishing unit.

Overall, this last example provides important insights into the necessity of a reliable and efficient model-based control strategy to increase the robustness of an integrated bioprocess based on perfusion cell culture, thus favoring its spreading in industrial settings.

## 4. Perfusion for intracellular products: Polyhydroxyalkanoates

Polyhydroxyalkanoates (PHA) are naturally occurring polymers, produced intracellularly by bacteria for carbon and energy storage. These polymers have the potential to replace conventional plastics, a reason that incentivized their research (Medeiros Garcia Alcântara et al., 2020). However, the adopted production processes, largely based on traditional batch technologies, limit the availability of these polymers and therefore hamper their success at the commercial scale.

To alleviate these drawbacks, a new type of continuous perfusion bioreactor for intracellular bioproducts was developed (see Fig. 7). This reactor features two outlets. One comes directly from the broth, containing the cells with the product. The other features a retention device which enables the achievement of very high cell densities and absolute control of the nutritional needs of the culture. This process is particularly well suited for the continuous high-cell density cultures for intracellular bioproducts, such as PHA, since it can increase productivity and titers while reducing the plant footprint.

The process starts with a first reactor (N-1 seed), where the cells are retained in the vessel through the retention device, allowing the achievement of very high cell densities. This stage is the start-up of the process. Then, the cells are transferred to the production bioreactor with two outlets,

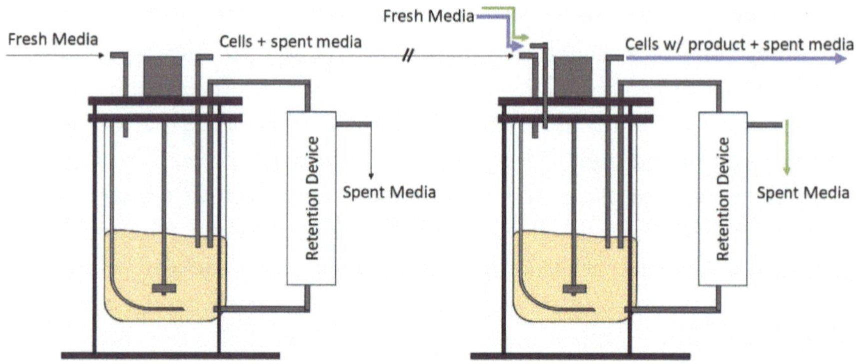


**Fig. 7** Schematic representation of the proposed perfusion-based process for intracellular products. The first reactor is a HD reactor working in fed-batch mode, which produces the high cell density inoculum for the second bioreactor. In this reactor, product accumulation occurs within the cells and the addition of fresh media can be freely controlled (green arrows) based on nutrient needs without having a wash-out of the cells. This is due to the constant flow rate of the stream containing the cells (blue arrows). (The symbol // indicates a discontinuous transfer.)

in which the cell-containing one operates at the maximum dilution rate. This rate is still limited by the cell growth rate, but since cell densities are higher than in traditional chemostats, the productivity is higher. Furthermore, a retention device is present also in this second bioreactor in order to obtain stable operation even at such high cell density values. This, in fact, allows the supply of enough nutrients to the reactor to maintain the very high density of cells. In this way, more media can be fed into the bioreactor while maintaining the bioreactor within stable operating conditions (see Fig. 7, blue arrows), since the media excess is removed via the permeate side of the retention device (see Fig. 7, green arrows).

The proposed perfusion-based continuous bioreactor has increased productivity by more than 45% compared to a fed-batch baseline process, while allowing for a stable process for more than 10 days (see Fig. 8). This application appears particularly promising, because its success requires the use of waste feedstocks (Brown, 2010), which have inherently low nutrient concentration and mostly low productivities. The proposed system has the potential to intensify and increase the productivities of these processes through the continuous operating mode.

Furthermore, this system can be adapted for the production of intracellular products which are not growth associated. In this case, the culture is run in two stages, a growth stage in which the cell density increases and a

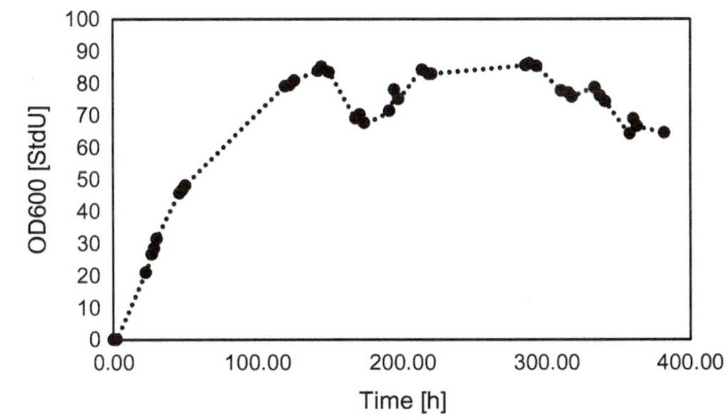


**Fig. 8** Cell density measured in terms of optical density at 600nm vs time for a single-stage perfusion bioreactor for the production of intracellular bioproducts, such as polyhydroxyalkanoates.

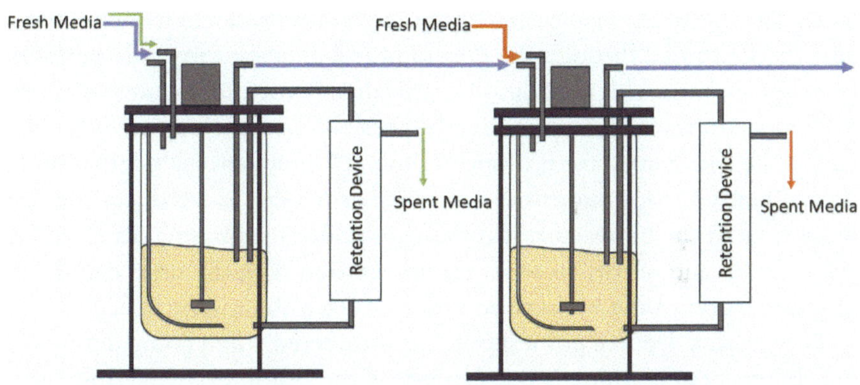


**Fig. 9** Schematic representation of a two-stage perfusion bioreactor system for the production of intracellular bioproducts which are not growth associated. In the first bioreactor the conditions are optimized for cellular growth, while in the second one for product accumulation.

production stage, in which the product is accumulated. Since the optimal process conditions for these stages might be different, research has been conducted into separating the two stages and having them occur in different but connected bioreactors (Atlić et al., 2011). An example is the production of polyhydroxyalkanoates using *Cupriavidus necator*, in which PHA accumulation is increased by the absence of nitrogen (Medeiros Garcia Alcântara et al., 2020). In this case, it is possible to implement two perfusion bioreactors operating continuously, each with its ideal fresh media supply (see Fig. 9).

## 5. Conclusions

The growing demand for biological products, which has been exacerbated by the COVID-19 pandemic for which more than 50% of the prescribed drugs are indeed biologics, stimulated already from the beginning of the century an intense research in converting conventional fermentation processes from batch to continuous. The simple CSTR configuration is not the ideal option for mammalian cell cultures, which is by far the most common expression system for complex products, such as therapeutic proteins. In fact, high flow rates of fresh media cannot be implemented in this configuration, due to the cell wash-out that this would induce.

A more efficient configuration brought to the attention is the perfusion bioreactor, which deviates from a CSTR by the addition of a cell retention device. This alleviates the concern related to the cell wash-out, allowing a drastic increase in the viable cell density and hence productivity. The advantages demonstrated through the development of laboratory-scale perfusion processes are manifold. In addition to the already mentioned increase in the productivity it is worth mentioning the possibility of reaching a steady-state, that can be maintained for prolonged time. This reduces the fluctuations of the product CQAs, uniforms the microenvironment and reduces the residence time in the bioreactor. It is then particularly promising for an industrial scale-up and in particular for the integration with the units deputed to the purification of the biologic in order to reach the market specifications.

However, a decisive point should be considered when going for continuous bioprocesses, which is the stability of the cell lines used. Most often, these cells undergo mutations that lead to a drift in the composition and titer of the harvest. It follows that the adoption of these processes on large production campaigns cannot disregard the development of a reliable and efficient control strategy, able to monitor in real time the product CQAs and intervene promptly at the level of the bioreactor operating conditions.

## References

Abu-Absi NR, Kenty BM, Cuellar ME, et al.: Real time monitoring of multiple parameters in mammalian cell culture bioreactors using an in-line Raman spectroscopy probe, *Biotechnol Bioeng* 108(5):1215–1221, 2011.

Angepat S, Gorenflo VM, Piret JM: Accelerating perfusion process optimization by scanning non-steady-state responses, *Biotechnol Bioeng* 92(4):472–478, 2005.

Atlić A, Koller M, Scherzer D, et al.: Continuous production of poly([R]-3-hydroxybutyrate) by Cupriavidus necator in a multistage bioreactor cascade, *Appl Microbiol Biotechnol* 91(2):295–304, 2011.

Bielser J-M, Domaradzki J, Souquet J, Morbidelli M, Broly H: Semi-continuous scale-down models for clone and operating parameter screening in perfusion bioreactors, *Biotechnol Prog* 35(3), 2019, e2790.
Bonham-Carter J, Shevitz J: A brief history of perfusion biomanufacturing, *Bioprocess Int*, 2011. http://www.bioprocessintl.com/upstream-processing/bioreactors/a-brief-history-of-perfusion-biomanufacturing-322322/.
Brown TA: *Introduction of DNA into living cells*, 2010.
Castilho LR, Medronho RA: Cell retention devices for suspended-cell perfusion cultures, In Schügerl K, Zeng A-P, Aunins JG, et al., editors: *Tools and applications of biochemical engineering science*, Berlin, Heidelberg, 2002, Springer Berlin Heidelberg, pp 129–169.
Chuppa S, Tsai Y-S, Yoon S, et al.: Fermentor temperature as a tool for control of high-density perfusion cultures of mammalian cells, *Biotechnol Bioeng* 55(2):328–338, 1997.
Clincke M-F, Mölleryd C, Zhang Y, Lindskog E, Walsh K, Chotteau V: Very high density of CHO cells in perfusion by ATF or TFF in WAVE bioreactor™. Part I. Effect of the cell density on the process, *Biotechnol Prog* 29(3):754–767, 2013.
Coffman J, Lin H, Wang S, et al.: Balancing continuous, integrated, and batch processing, In *Integrated continuous biomanufacturing III*, 2017.
Croughan MS, Konstantinov KB, Cooney C: The future of industrial bioprocessing: batch or continuous? *Biotechnol Bioeng* 112(4):648–651, 2015.
Diallo BK, Riffard C, Le Gouge K, Teillaud JL: MAbs: the history of a basic research or the curiosity as a source of wealth, *Med Sci (Paris)* 35(12):926–936, 2020.
Doran PM: *Bioprocess engineering principles*, 1995, Academic Press.
Dowd JE, Jubb A, Kwok KE, Piret JM: Optimization and control of perfusion cultures using a viable cell probe and cell specific perfusion rates, *Cytotechnology* 42(1):35–45, 2003.
EMA: *International conference on harmonisation of technical requirements for registration of pharmaceuticals for human use, Q8(R2)—pharmaceutical development*, 2009.
Europa AF, Gambhir A, Fu P-C, Hu W-S: Multiple steady states with distinct cellular metabolism in continuous culture of mammalian cells, *Biotechnol Bioeng* 67(1):25–34, 2000.
FDA: *International conference on harmonisation of technical requirements for registration of pharmaceuticals for human use, Q11—development and manufacture of drug substances (chemical entities and biotechnological/biological entities)*, 2012.
Feidl F, Vogg S, Wolf M, et al.: Process-wide control and automation of an integrated continuous manufacturing platform for antibodies, *Biotechnol Bioeng* 117(5): 1367–1380, 2020.
Fernandez-de-Cossio-Diaz J, Leon K, Mulet R: Characterizing steady states of genome-scale metabolic networks in continuous cell cultures, *PLOS Comput Biol* 13(11):1–22, 2017.
Godawat R, Konstantinov K, Rohani M, Warikoo V: End-to-end integrated fully continuous production of recombinant monoclonal antibodies, *J Biotechnol* 213:13–19, 2015.
Gouveia FF, Rahbek JP, Mortensen AR, et al.: Using PAT to accelerate the transition to continuous API manufacturing, *Anal Bioanal Chem* 409(3):821–832, 2017.
Hu W-S: Overview of cell culture technology, In *Cell culture bioprocess engineering*, 2012a.
Hu W-S: Cell retention and perfusion, In *Cell culture bioprocess engineering*, 2012b, pp 249–262.
Janoschek S, Schulze M, Zijlstra G, Greller G, Matuszczyk J: A protocol to transfer a fed-batch platform process into semi-perfusion mode: the benefit of automated small-scale bioreactors compared to shake flasks as scale-down model, *Biotechnol Prog* 35(2), 2019, e2757.
Jin L, Wang ZS, Cao Y, Sun RQ, Zhou H, Cao RY: Establishment and optimization of a high-throughput mimic perfusion model in ambr® 15, *Biotechnol Lett* 43(2): 423–433, 2021.
Jungbauer A, Hammerschmidt N, Khinast J, Rantanen J: Integrated continuous manufacturing of biopharmaceuticals, In Kleinebudde P, editor: *Continuous manufacturing of pharmaceuticals*, Chichester, UK, 2017, John Wiley & Sons, Ltd, pp 247–281.
Kaplon H, Reichert JM: Antibodies to watch in 2021, *mAbs* 13(1):1860476, 2021.

Karst DJ, Serra E, Villiger TK, Soos M, Morbidelli M: Characterization comparison of ATF and TFF in stirred bioreactors for continuous mammalian cell culture processes, *Biochem Eng J* 110:17–26, 2016.
Karst DJ, Steinebach F, Soos M, Morbidelli M: Process performance and product quality in an integrated continuous antibody production process, *Biotechnol Bioeng* 114(2):298–307, 2017a.
Karst DJ, Steinhoff RF, Kopp MRG, et al.: Intracellular CHO cell metabolite profiling reveals steady-state dependent metabolic fingerprints in perfusion culture, *Biotechnol Prog* 33(4):879–890, 2017b.
Karst DJ, Steinebach F, Morbidelli M: Continuous integrated manufacturing of therapeutic proteins, *Curr Opin Biotechnol* 53:76–84, 2018.
Konstantinov KB, Cooney CL: White paper on continuous bioprocessing May 20–21, 2014 continuous manufacturing symposium, *J Pharm Sci* 104(3):813–820, 2015.
Konstantinov KB, Tsai Y, Moles D, Matanguihan R: Control of long-term perfusion Chinese hamster ovary cell culture by glucose auxostat, *Biotechnol Prog* 12(1):100–109, 1996.
Konstantinov K, Goudar C, Ng M, et al.: The 'push-to-low' approach for optimization of high-density perfusion cultures of animal cells, *Adv Biochem Eng Biotechnol* 101:75–98, 2006.
Medeiros Garcia Alcântara J, Distante F, Storti G, Moscatelli D, Morbidelli M, Sponchioni M: Current trends in the production of biodegradable bioplastics: the case of polyhydroxyalkanoates, *Biotechnol Adv* 42:107582, 2020.
Myerson AS, Krumme M, Nasr M, Thomas H, Braatz RD: Control systems engineering in continuous pharmaceutical manufacturing May 20–21, 2014 continuous manufacturing symposium, *J Pharm Sci* 104(3):832–839, 2015.
Narayanan H, Sponchioni M, Morbidelli M: Integration and digitalization in the manufacturing of therapeutic proteins, *Chem Eng Sci* 248, 2022, 117159.
Ozturk SS, Thrift JC, Blackie JD, Naveh D: Real-time monitoring and control of glucose and lactate concentrations in a mammalian cell perfusion reactor, *Biotechnol Bioeng* 53(4):372–378, 1997.
Teixeira AP, Oliveira R, Alves PM, Carrondo MJT: Advances in on-line monitoring and control of mammalian cell cultures: supporting the PAT initiative, *Biotechnol Adv* 27(6):726–732, 2009.
Voisard D, Meuwly F, Ruffieux P-A, Baer G, Kadouri A: Potential of cell retention techniques for large-scale high-density perfusion culture of suspended mammalian cells, *Biotechnol Bioeng* 82(7):751–765, 2003.
Wang S, Godfrey S, Ravikrishnan J, Lin H, Vogel J, Coffman J: Shear contributions to cell culture performance and product recovery in ATF and TFF perfusion systems, *J Biotechnol* 246:52–60, 2017.
Warikoo V, Godawat R, Brower K, et al.: Integrated continuous production of recombinant therapeutic proteins, *Biotechnol Bioeng* 109(12):3018–3029, 2012.
Wolf MKF, Lorenz V, Karst DJ, Souquet J, Broly H, Morbidelli M: Development of a shake-tube-based scale-down model for perfusion cultures, *Biotechnol Bioeng*, 2018.
Wolf M, Bielser J-M, Morbidelli M: *Perfusion cell culture processes for biopharmaceuticals*, 2020, Cambridge University Press.
Woodside SM, Bowen BD, Piret JM: Mammalian cell retention devices for stirred perfusion bioreactors, *Cytotechnology* 28(1–3):163–175, 1998.
Xu S, Chen H: High-density mammalian cell cultures in stirred-tank bioreactor without external pH control, *J Biotechnol* 231:149–159, 2016.
Xu S, Gavin J, Jiang R, Chen H: Bioreactor productivity and media cost comparison for different intensified cell culture processes, *Biotechnol Prog* 33(4):867–878, 2017.

CHAPTER TWO

# Continuous countercurrent chromatography for the downstream processing of bioproducts: A focus on flow-through technologies

**Ismaele Fioretti, Tae Keun Kim, and Mattia Sponchioni***
Department of Chemistry, Materials and Chemical Engineering "Giulio Natta," Politecnico di Milano, Milano, Italy
*Corresponding author: e-mail address: mattia.sponchioni@polimi.it

## Contents



## Abstract

The necessity of ensuring consistent purity for satisfying the high standards required from biopharmaceutical companies led the liquid chromatography to become the gold standard for the downstream purification of biotherapeutics. The possibility of switching between different resins and buffer combinations allows to successfully perform separations of structurally similar molecules by exploiting peculiar properties of the product, including: conformation, charge, hydrophobicity and size. However, underutilization of the resin, low productivity and poor product recovery when aiming at an imposed purity of the product pool have been intrinsic limitations of the single-column batch chromatography. To tackle these drawbacks, multi-column continuous countercurrent operations have been introduced in the field and have become effective solutions to improve the performances of the downstream

*Advances in Chemical Engineering*, Volume 59
ISSN 0065-2377
https://doi.org/10.1016/bs.ache.2022.03.002

processing of biopharmaceuticals. Nowadays, most of the new technologies, for both capture and polishing processes, exploit the simulated moving bed (SMB) strategy for the operational configuration. In this chapter, the concepts behind the SMB and the different continuous chromatographic techniques based on the frontal mode, which have been demonstrated successful in the purification of biologics ensuring high yield and productivity, are discussed. In particular, the working principles of each technique are explained in detail, together with some case studies reported to compare their process performances with those obtained with a single-column operation. Finally, a critical presentation of the perspectives of these techniques and the gap still to be covered to reach industrial maturity is introduced.

# 1. Introduction

## 1.1 Basic principles of chromatography for biotherapeutics

In the drug development, the active principles are traditionally classified based on their molecular weight into small and large molecules. Small molecule drugs, with a molecular weight not exceeding 900 g/mol, have been dominant so far, as more than 90% of the current on-the-market drugs fall into this category (De la Torre and Albericio, 2018; Narayanan et al., 2022; Nuventra Pharma Sciences, 2020; Rader, 2008; Rufer, 2021; Walsh, 2018). Their small size and physiochemical properties allow to be effective enzyme inhibitors and allosteric modifiers (De la Torre and Albericio, 2018; Rader, 2008; Rufer, 2021; Veber et al., 2002; Walsh, 2018). While the development of small molecules continues, the new advancement of recombinant DNA technology and protein engineering in the last few decades has enabled the synthesis of large molecules from transformed microorganisms or transfected animal cells (De la Torre and Albericio, 2018; Makurvet, 2021). These biotherapeutics proved to be highly specific, showing a higher affinity and lower toxicity compared to their small molecule counterparts. This justifies the exponential growth in the interest and clinical research that these molecules are attracting. As a matter of fact, during the Covid-19 pandemic, 53% out of all considered treatments were biologics (Narayanan et al., 2022). This number further increases if we consider that the majority of vaccines approved against Covid-19 are based on mRNA.

Biologics are characterized by a relatively large size, ranging from 3,000 to 150,000 Da and thus exhibit more structural complexity than small molecules. Among them, different species are included, *i.e.*, monoclonal antibodies, peptides, fusion proteins, vaccines, hormones and oligonucleotides. Most of them are recombinantly produced from bacteria such as *E. coli* or more from mammalian cells in those cases where post-translational modifications are important to achieve the therapeutic action. In this case, Chinese Hamster Ovary (CHO) cells are the most common expression system (De la Torre and Albericio, 2018; Makurvet, 2021). These microorganisms produce the required biotherapeutic together with additional molecules required for the cell survival, including DNA, host-cell proteins (HCP), endonucleases. This broad family of species represent the so-called process-related impurities that need to be separated from the target molecule. In addition, given the structural complexity and process sensitivity, the complete characterization of large molecules is often difficult to achieve, and molecularly similar variants of the product are typically produced (Makurvet, 2021; Mallik et al., 2016; Rader, 2008). These impurities include isomers, charge variants, different glycoforms and molecules with different chain length. These molecules, are often referred to as product-related impurities and their separation is particularly challenging, given the similarity to the product. To ensure consistent purity for satisfying the high biomedical market standards, liquid chromatography is extensively employed as its potential has been proved for decades (Carta and Jungbauer, 2010; Coskun, 2016; Mallik et al., 2016).

Liquid chromatography has become an indispensable separation technique for purification and identification in processing large molecules. As each molecule exhibits its own charge, size, shape, and hydrophobicity, one or more characteristics can be selected to design the most suitable chromatographic technique allowing the separation of the product from both process-related and product-related impurities (Mallik et al., 2016). For efficient purification and analysis, a fixed bed adsorbent, or stationary phase, and a liquid mobile phase need to be chosen following the means of separation and corresponding characteristics of the target molecule (Carta and Jungbauer, 2010; Coskun, 2016; Pfister et al., 2018). In the conventional chromatography, the differential partitioning of the molecules comprised in a mixture between the mobile phase and the stationary phase allows them to be separated according to the molecule affinity to the chromatographic resin, which is converted in a different elution time (Carta and Jungbauer, 2010; Coskun, 2016; Pfister et al., 2018).

## 1.2 Types of chromatography

A type of chromatography is selected based on the expected differences between the properties of the target molecule and those of the impurities.

The four properties in a biotherapeutic that are typically exploited for the separation are charge, size, hydrophobicity, and shape (Mallik et al., 2016). After selecting a property of the target to investigate, general chromatographic steps are involved with appropriate buffer preparation. These steps include equilibration, load feed, wash, elution and clean-in-place (CIP). The equilibration of the stationary phase allows the elimination of eventual storage chemicals, or storage buffers, as well as the restoration of the binding sites for adsorption of the molecules in the mixture to be separated. In the load feed, the product and other species are adsorbed on the stationary phase and get concentrated on the resin, while unadsorbed species flow through the column without retention (Carta and Jungbauer, 2010; Coskun, 2016; Pfister et al., 2018). The wash step allows eluting any residual unadsorbed species in the column or very weakly adsorbed species using the same equilibration buffer or a similar buffer (Coskun, 2016). The elution introduces a modifier in the system with a sufficient concentration to desorb and then elute the adsorbed species. The CIP completely removes any strongly adsorbed species or other contaminants that remain after the elution step. This is necessary to ensure the full binding capacity and high resolution of the column is restored in a subsequent run of the chromatography. In general, as clean-in-place, or regeneration, buffers are chemically harsh for the stationary phase and thus not suitable for long-term storage, removing the regeneration buffer and substituting it with an appropriate storage buffer to prevent microbial growth and/or salt precipitation is necessary by the addition of a storage step (Mallik et al., 2016). In case of successive runs, the storage step is not required as the last step of each cycle and can replaced by re-equilibration of the column.

### *1.2.1 Ion exchange chromatography*

Ion exchange chromatography is one of the most frequently used chromatographic mode for purification of biologics, as it can separate different molecular species that exhibit only minor charge differences from each other (Carta and Jungbauer, 2010; Coskun, 2016; Pfister et al., 2018). As each large molecule is composed of its own unique sequence of amino acids or nucleobases for oligonucleotides, a unique net surface charge at a given pH for each large molecule is expected. Ion exchange chromatography exploits the relationship between net surface charge and pH to create reversible electrostatic attraction of charged molecules to the stationary phase, which has covalently attached side groups of opposite charges, to achieve separation between each species (Fritz, 2004). To properly design an ion exchange chromatography, the concept of isoelectric point (pI) is essential.

This applies in particular to poly(amino acids), few of them exhibiting weak acidic or weak alkaline residues. Then, for a biologic, the pI is defined as the value of pH at which the net charge of the molecule goes to zero (Carta and Jungbauer, 2010; Coskun, 2016; Pfister et al., 2018). Molecules with pI higher than the biological pH (*i.e.*, 7.4) show a net positive charge in physiological conditions, and then bind to negatively-charged media, or cation exchangers. On the other hand, those showing a lower pI, preferentially bind to anion exchangers (Carta and Jungbauer, 2010; Coskun, 2016; Pfister et al., 2018).

In ion exchange chromatography, pH and ionic strength of the equilibration, feed load, wash, and elution buffers play critical roles in designing binding and elution profiles of the chromatography (Carta and Jungbauer, 2010; Coskun, 2016; Pfister et al., 2018). From the equilibration to wash steps, pH is selected to design not only which type of the ion exchangers is used but also the degree of its binding affinity to the designed exchanger, as the larger difference between pI of the product and pH of the buffers allows the target to be adsorbed more strongly. Ionic strength, which expresses the effect of counterions, such as sodium or chloride, is another crucial parameter for a buffer used in ion exchange chromatography (Carta and Jungbauer, 2010; Coskun, 2016; Pfister et al., 2018). In particular, increasing the ionic strength introduces more counterions to compete with the charged groups on the biomolecule for binding on the stationary phase, as well as reduces the extension of the electrical double layer on both the biologics and the resin, thus allowing the desorption of the adsorbed species. Therefore, while low ionic strength buffers are used during the loading step to favor the adsorption, in the elution step the ionic strength is altered to desorb the adsorbed species, including the target. The adsorbed species with the lowest net charge are eluted first and the ones with the highest net charge last (Carta and Jungbauer, 2010; Coskun, 2016; Pfister et al., 2018). Similarly, changing pH to neutralize net charges of the adsorbed species elutes the lowest net charge first. From this description, it appears that ion exchange chromatography is particularly suitable for the separation of charge variants, functionalized proteins and oligonucleotides and for all the cases where a slight variation of the charged groups between the product and the impurities can be leveraged.

### 1.2.2 Size exclusion chromatography

Size exclusion chromatography, or gel filtration, separates molecules based on their size as they pass through pores of the stationary phase (Carta and Jungbauer, 2010; Wang et al., 2010). The stationary phase consists of spherical beads with different pore sizes. The portion of these pores that is accessible to the molecules in the mobile phase is mainly determined by their size and shape, while no specific adsorption occurs, unlike other chromatographic modes (Malik and Pasch, 2021; Wang et al., 2010). The lack of the adsorptive properties simplifies the steps of purification, in which equilibration, load feed, and wash steps are operated. As all molecules in the feed flow-through with interaction-free diffusion with the stationary phase and the separation is based on the peculiar size, the elution step is typically not required (Carta and Jungbauer, 2010; Wang et al., 2010).

In size exclusion chromatography, the resolution is governed by three factors, which are the feed volume, buffer, and pore size of the stationary phase (Wang et al., 2010). A feed volume lower than 2% of the column volume is recommended to ensure the maximum resolution but up to 5% may be acceptable depending on the required separation (Carta and Jungbauer, 2010). Therefore, the limitation on the feed volume can be alleviated by increasing the column volume or by concentrating the feed before injection (Malik and Pasch, 2021). In general, isocratic elution is used for the separation, which will be discussed in detail in Section 1.3.2 (Carta and Jungbauer, 2010). The buffer components are selected in order to reduce the non-specific or weak electrostatic interactions between the feed and the medium. This is typically achieved by adding a low concentration of electrolytes to prevent instability of the feed during the separation (Carta and Jungbauer, 2010). Choosing an appropriate molecular weight cut-off (MWCO) of the pores ensures the discrimination of the size of the target with other species. MWCO is a semi-quantitative way of specifying the size of the pores, typically in terms of membrane filtration, but is also a characteristic that represents the stationary phase of the technique (Malik and Pasch, 2021). Molecules that have higher molecular weight than the MWCO fails to permeate the pores and then cannot be separated on that particular resin (Malik and Pasch, 2021). Using this characteristic, buffer exchange, or desalting, is possible by leveraging on the molecular weight difference between the product and salt/buffer molecules (Carta and Jungbauer, 2010; Pfister et al., 2018). This step is used to exchange the buffer of the process intermediate before injecting as the load feed of a subsequent chromatography or after chromatography at its storage condition. In the buffer exchange, the difference between the two species is usually very large and an overlap of the two species is less likely, thus allowing larger feed volumes up to 30% of the column volume (Carta and Jungbauer, 2010; Malik and Pasch, 2021).

### 1.2.3 Hydrophobic interaction chromatography

Hydrophobic interaction chromatography (HIC) separates large molecules based on their surface hydrophobicity (Carta and Jungbauer, 2010). Driven by van der Waals forces between hydrophobic regions of the molecules and the stationary phase, the interaction is modulated by the addition of salt (Carta and Jungbauer, 2010; Pfister et al., 2018). As opposed to a "normal phase" chromatography, which uses hydrophilic interaction between large molecules and the stationary phase, this technique exploits the different hydrophobicity of the molecules to be separated (Pfister et al., 2018). In general, the feed is loaded at high ionic strength, which reduces the solvation of the target and other species in the feed, and, as solvation is reduced, hydrophobic regions are more exposed, allowing the molecule adsorption to the stationary phase. Decreasing the salt concentration desorbs the adsorbed species from the stationary phase and, in order of increasing hydrophobicity, elution takes place (Carta and Jungbauer, 2010; McCue, 2009; Pfister et al., 2018).

In HIC, four factors mainly affect the design and the performance of the separation, which are the ligands of the stationary phase, the ionic strength and pH of the mobile phase, and temperature (McCue, 2009). The ligand determines not only the strength of the hydrophobic interaction but also the types of mobile phases that should be used. Grafted on cross-linked agarose or synthetic copolymers, the ligands of HIC media are characterized by either alkyl chains or aryl groups (Carta and Jungbauer, 2010; Pfister et al., 2018). The interactions can be modulated by the addition of a salt. Depending on which type of ion in a salt, it can increase or decrease the strength of the interactions (Carta and Jungbauer, 2010; McCue, 2009; Pfister et al., 2018). If anti-chaotropic ions, of which include phosphate and sulfate for anions, and ammonium, potassium, sodium for cations, are prevalent, hydrophobic interactions and protein precipitation by salting-out are promoted (Carta and Jungbauer, 2010). In fact, preferential binding of the anti-chaotropic ions to water outcompetes water-large molecule interaction and thus decreases the wetted area and solubility, promoting intermolecular interaction (McCue, 2009). Therefore, at a high concentration of anti-chaotropic ions, large molecules are adsorbed on the stationary phase (McCue, 2009). To elute the adsorbed species, the salt concentration is decreased to promote stabilizing effects and decrease their hydrophobicity (McCue, 2009). Conversely, increasing chaotropic ions, of which anions include nitrate, iodide, bromide, and cations include calcium, barium, magnesium, promotes salting-in, which solubilizes large molecules and decreases their binding to the medium (McCue, 2009). The pH of the mobile phases can be an important factor affecting hydrophobic interactions. As the pH deviates further from the pI of large molecules, increased charges of the biologic decrease hydrophobicity. It is found that the binding behavior of large molecules shifts drastically when pH values are below 5 and above 8.5 (Andjelković et al., 2017). Although this effect can vary as each large molecule has different pI and can interact differently with different salts, pH can be introduced as another variable when designing HIC (Andjelković et al., 2017; Pfister et al., 2018).

The affinity of hydrophobic interactions has a temperature dependency (McCue, 2009). As the change of temperature affects structure and solubility of large molecules, the interaction may shift. Even though the role of temperature in HIC is not completely understood, in general, increasing temperature in HIC promotes the interaction, and lowering temperature promotes elution (McCue, 2009).

### 1.2.4 Reversed-phase chromatography

Compared to HIC, reversed-phase chromatography (RPC) still exploits hydrophobic interactions to promote the separation of the molecules in a mixture. However, in this case the stationary phase is more hydrophobic (Pfister et al., 2018). Characterized by alkyl chains, which are C4, C8, or C18 in length grafted on silica backbones, the ligand of RPC strongly adsorbs the hydrophobic regions of large molecules and thus its elution or reversion requires using non-polar, organic solvents (Pfister et al., 2018). The polarity of the mobile phase is modulated by the addition of the organic solvents. Decreasing the polarity of the mobile phase by increasing the organic solvent percentage allows for elution of the adsorbed species in order of increasing hydrophobicity. Incompatibility of large molecules in organic solvents that can cause unfolding and aggregation hinders using RPC for biologics, but the technique is suitable for small molecules, such as peptides.

### 1.2.5 Affinity chromatography

Affinity chromatography (AC) involves specific interactions between active sites on the exposed surface of the biotherapeutics and a specific ligand anchored to the stationary phase (Carta and Jungbauer, 2010; Pfister et al., 2018). In AC, van der Waals forces, hydrophobic, electrostatic interactions, and hydrogen bonds are used for its high specificity (Carta and Jungbauer, 2010; Pfister et al., 2018). The interactions can be biospecific, which can be used for the purification of enzymes, hormones, antibodies, nucleic acids, and specific molecules, or non-biospecific. In this case, the most applied technique is the metal affinity chromatography (MAC), which exploits the interaction between transition metals including copper, zinc, nickel, or iron and metal-binding sites of large molecules, mainly histidine residues (Pfister et al., 2018). Due to its high selectivity, AC is used as the first capture step, followed by other polishing steps to improve purity, and further remove any impurity (Freitag, 1998; Hagel et al., 2008; Mukherjee, 2019). In the current biopharmaceuticals, Protein A affinity resin is most frequently used for the purification of recombinant monoclonal antibodies. It consists of five immunoglobulin-binding domains, which are most suitable for binding immunoglobulin G (IgG) at the heavy chain of the Fc region with high specificity (Andjelković et al., 2017; Pfister et al., 2018).

Although AC is an ideal technique that provides a high degree of purification and yield in a single step, several drawbacks are raised, which are its cost and stability (De Luca et al., 2020). Coupling ligands to the stationary phase may require expensive and hazardous chemicals and are destabilized readily by elution or CIP conditions (Hagel et al., 2008; Poole, 2003). The destabilized linkage is easily disrupted, resulting in ligand leaching. For example, leaching of Protein A ligands in the elution phase will result in co-elution with the target (Hagel et al., 2008; Poole, 2003). The leached Protein A ligands must be detected and quantified to satisfy a critical quality control step in the production process (Carta and Jungbauer, 2010; Hagel et al., 2008; Poole, 2003). In the case of the detection of leaching, it must be removed through further polishing steps, using other chromatographic methods, such as IEX or HIC (Hagel et al., 2008).

AC that uses non-biospecific binding is called immobilized metal affinity chromatography (IMAC) (Pfister et al., 2018). The most used IMAC technique is His-tag purification. A strong binding between histidine-tagged recombinant large molecules, or large molecules with surface-exposed histidine groups, and immobilized copper or nickel ions on the stationary phase can show an intermediate selectivity between AC and IEC, depending on the number of the histidine groups exposed on the surface of the molecule (Pfister et al., 2018). Its elution can be achieved by decreasing pH, introducing competitive ligands such as imidazole, or adding a chelating agent. Despite its simplicity, IMAC is not readily used in industry. Recombination of His tags may interrupt a native conformation of large molecules that can decrease the biological functions, and its cleavage by enzymatic or chemical reaction require introduction of another purification step (Pfister et al., 2018).

## 1.3 Mode of operations

If we consider a mixture comprising two molecules A and B that is fed to a chromatographic column (Fig. 1A), with A being the more weakly adsorbed species and B the more strongly adsorbed molecule, different operations can be conducted for their separation, irrespectively of the stationary phase used. These operations, described in detailed in the following, are based on specific durations and programs of the load and elution phases, with the latter that may involve the addition of a particular modifier.

### *1.3.1 Displacement chromatography*

The displacement chromatography makes use of a displacer, which is a modifier with a higher affinity to the stationary phase than any species in the feed, to competitively bind to the active sites of the resin, thus replacing and favoring the desorption of the species to be separated (Carta and Jungbauer, 2010). This desorption rate is inversely proportional to the affinity of a molecule to the sites of the resin. In Fig. 1B, the less strongly adsorbed specie A in the load feed migrates faster through the column, while the more strongly adsorbed specie B follows, thus each upstream specie acts as a displacer for each specie at its immediate downstream, and finally eluted by the addition of the displacer (D) (Carta and Jungbauer, 2010). These consecutive zones of separated species are called a displacement train, as shown in Fig. 1B (Carta and Jungbauer, 2010; Freitag, 1998). In the elution phase, all species are eluted in order of increasing affinity, followed by the displacer, at the same linear velocity. Using the technique, with minor or unknown difference in affinity, the separation is easy to achieve (Carta and Jungbauer, 2010; Freitag, 1998). Although the technique is well established to separate inorganic and organic low-molecular weight molecules, candidates for suitable displacers for large molecule separation are difficult to find in terms of reusability of the stationary phase, cost, and toxicity (Freitag, 1998).

### *1.3.2 Elution chromatography*

The concept of elution chromatography (EC) is based on the introduction of a chemical modifier in the mobile phase that desorbs the species from the chromatographic resin (Carta and Jungbauer, 2010; Pfister et al., 2018). This modifier exhibits lower affinity to the stationary phase than the species comprised in the mixture. The low modifier concentration allows non-specific binding impurities to flow through the stationary phase (Berruex and Freitag, 2003; Carta and Jungbauer, 2010; Pfister et al., 2018). The desorption is dependent

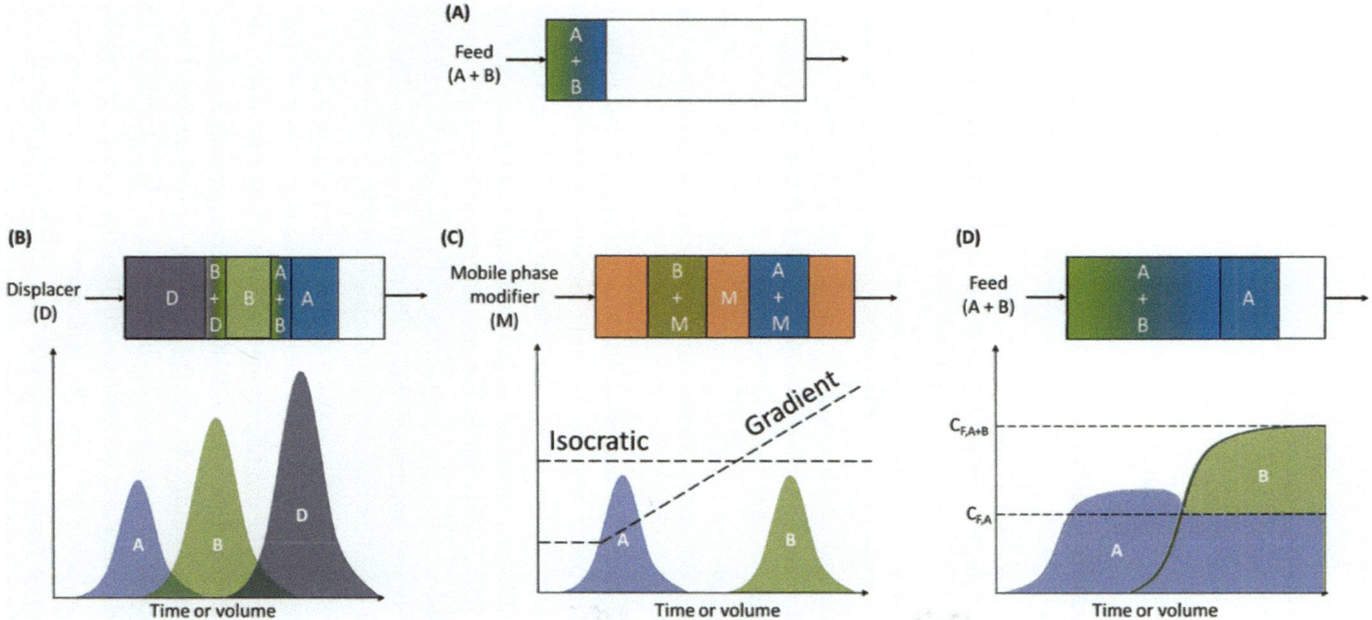


**Fig. 1** Schematic representation of (A) load feed of the three modes of operation, (B) displacement chromatography, (C) elution chromatography, and (D) frontal chromatography. From (B) to (D). Each mode of operation is shown with the distribution of all species in a chromatographic column and illustrative chromatogram.

on the molecule affinity at a local modifier concentration, and this can be modulated by two modes: isocratic elution and gradient elution, illustrated in the chromatogram of Fig. 1C. Isocratic elution uses a constant modifier concentration throughout the elution phase, while gradient elution varies the modifier concentration over time (Carta and Jungbauer, 2010; Pfister et al., 2018).

Isocratic elution is a suitable elution mode for analysis, especially for SEC. In this mode, the feed amount is kept low to ensure the robustness of the elution profile (Malik and Pasch, 2021; Wang et al., 2010). At low loadings, each species in the feed flows through the column independent of other species and thus is eluted at its unique retention time. However, when the feed amount exceeds the limit, the adsorption equilibrium becomes non-linear, and thus the bound species interact with each other, resulting in shifting of the retention time depending on the feed concentration (Carta and Jungbauer, 2010; Wang et al., 2010). Moreover, an inefficient separation is observed when the feed consists of species of widely different affinities to the stationary phase. As the modifier concentration is constant, weakly bound species are eluted with little or no separation, and strongly bound species are eluted very late or not eluted at all, leading to increased consumption of the mobile phase and inefficient operating time.

On the other hand, gradient elution can separate the feed as the modifier concentration can be controlled. A steady increase or abrupt increase of the modifier concentration in the mobile phase can elute the weakly bound species at a low modifier concentration, achieving a good separation from other species, and the strongly bound species at a high modifier concentration, that shortens the residence time of the species and enhances the productivity of the process (Carta and Jungbauer, 2010; Pfister et al., 2018). Therefore, the separation is not based on time but on the local modifier concentration. The steady increase of the modifier concentration is typically managed with a linear function of the time, so it is referred to as linear gradient elution (LGE), in which the slope of the modifier concentration is constant over time (Carta and Jungbauer, 2010; Pfister et al., 2018). It offers acceptable separations that minimize band broadening. An abrupt increase of the modifier concentration, or step gradient elution, is most challenging and yet useful at large scale when optimized (Carta and Jungbauer, 2010; Pfister et al., 2018). Step gradient elution can achieve complete separation of each species in narrow bands as its eluting modifier concentration can be reached in a series of isocratic steps, leading to shorter time compared to LGE.

### 1.3.3 *Frontal chromatography*

Frontal chromatography is characterized by the continuous loading of the feed in an appropriate mobile phase to favor the adsorption of all species but the target (Carta and Jungbauer, 2010; Pfister et al., 2018). In the feed load, competitive adsorption takes place as the stationary phase reaches its full capacity (Carta and Jungbauer, 2010; Pfister et al., 2018). Therefore, the least adsorbed species, which is designed to be the target, is obtained in pure form in the flow-through of the feed load, and, upon saturation of the column, other species will be desorbed in order of increasing affinity to the stationary phase (Kasai, 2014). As one could see, this technique contrasts with elution chromatography and resembles displacement chromatography. While in elution chromatography, the adsorption of the target is favored in the feed load and its elution can be achieved by applying an appropriate modifier concentration, the target is not adsorbed or the least strongly adsorbed to the stationary phase and thus is collected in the flow-through of the load feed in frontal chromatography. In displacement chromatography, an additional mobile phase containing the displacer is required to replace the adsorbed species, but only continuous load of the feed is required as the most strongly adsorbed species will act as "displacer" in frontal chromatography (Andjelković et al., 2017; Carta and Jungbauer, 2010). This technique is best suited for a binary separation, in which all impurities are designed to be adsorbed and the target is unretained in the stationary phase. In practice, the column is loaded before reaching the breakthrough of the impurities, washed using the same mobile phase of the feed to further collect the target in the interstitial voids, and finally regenerated (Andjelković et al., 2017; Carta and Jungbauer, 2010). In case of the unretained target in the load feed, the target is recovered at near or equal initial concentration of the feed. In Fig. 1D, an illustration of a continuous load feed is shown, in which the weakly adsorbed target (A) is concentrated by the competitive adsorption of the strongly adsorbed molecule (B) that allows A to form a pure component band. Due to the concentration occurring during this process, investigation of aggregation tendency or limited solubility is necessary to avoid any operational difficulties.

## 2. Continuous countercurrent chromatography

The general concept of a countercurrent separation is schematically illustrated in Fig. 2. We consider at first to have a column with a continuous flow of both stationary and mobile phases, occurring in opposite directions.

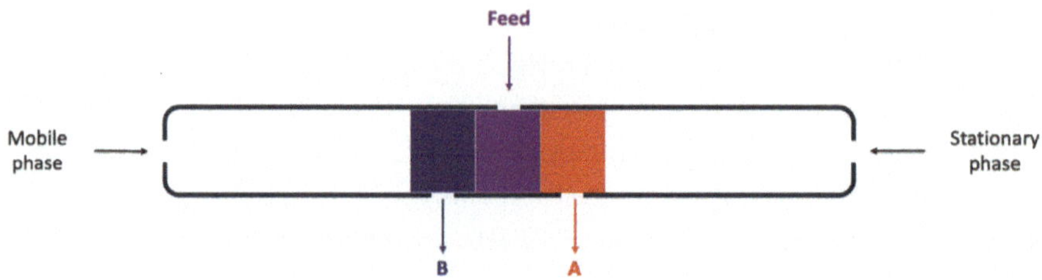


**Fig. 2** Binary separation with countercurrent movement of mobile and stationary phases.

Then, we inject in the column a binary mixture with the component A having a higher affinity to the mobile phase and the component B a higher affinity to the stationary phase. Once the column is fed, due to these different affinities of the species, the relative velocity between the mobile and the stationary phases can be adjusted so that the component A moves towards the mobile phase direction and the component B towards the stationary phase flow. In this way, the separation of the two species could be easily reached collecting both streams in two different outlets. Moreover, the driving force that moves the species from the liquid to the solid resin and vice versa is the difference in concentration of the compounds between the two phases: exploiting the countercurrent movement of the two phases this delta can be preserved over a more extended concentration gradient than for a hypothetical cocurrent mode of operation, thus allowing a more effective mass transport.

Since this countercurrent movement of the stationary phase and the mobile phase is complex to be achieved on real chromatographic setups, it is only simulated by exploiting more than one column, and changing the flow path of the chromatograph through the appropriate switching of valves. The concept of chromatographic purification exploiting multi-column simulated countercurrent adsorption units was first introduced in the 1960s for the purification of p-xylene from a mixture of aromatics on a Y-zeolite stationary phase and since then it is known as simulated moving bed (SMB) (Broughton, 1984; Broughton and Gerhold, 1961; Carta and Jungbauer, 2010; Juza et al., 2000; Yang et al., 2004). Although this technique was originally applied to hydrocarbon separations and more recently to chiral separations, most of the known continuous chromatographic technologies for the purification of biologics are based on this fundamental concept. As illustrated in Fig. 3, the practical implementation of the SMB is obtained dividing the system in four zones, each one comprising at least one fixed bed. In this

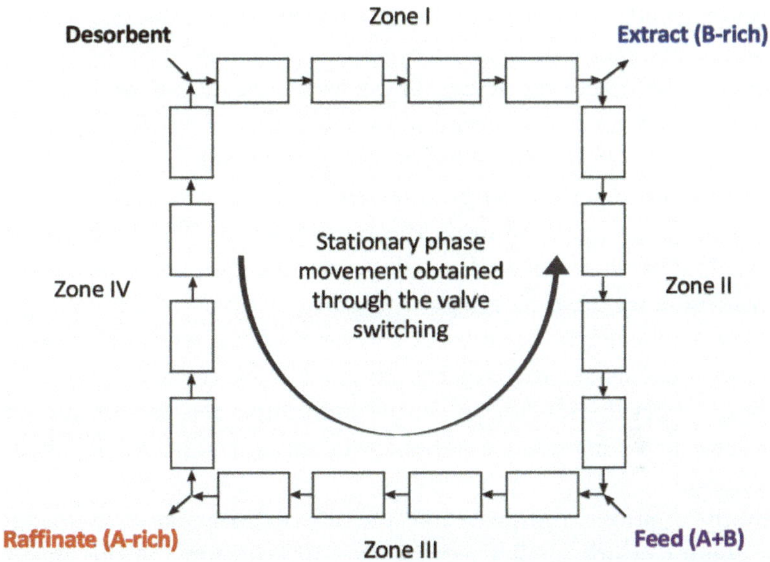


**Fig. 3** Scheme of the operational units implemented for the SMB. It consists of four zones, in this case each zone comprises four fixed beds. The feed is composed of a binary mixture of component A, with a higher affinity to the mobile phase, and a component B, with a higher affinity to the stationary phase.

schematic illustration, the feed, which is injected between zone II and zone III, contains a compound which has more affinity to the mobile phase (component A) and a specie with more affinity to the stationary phase (component B). The mobile phase moves clockwise from one zone to the next one, and the stationary phase proceeds in the opposite direction counterclockwise. Experimentally, this is obtained by switching the valve position in a way that each zone scales down by one position and the adsorbent is recycled from zone I to zone IV. Once the feed is injected, the component A is collected in the raffinate stream and the component B is collected in the extract stream. The main functions of each zone can be summarized as follows:

- Zone I desorbs the component B letting the adsorbent to be recycled in zone IV.
- Zone II desorbs the component A adsorbing at the same time the component B.
- Zone III adsorbs the component B allowing the component A to flow through.
- Zone IV adsorbs the component A.

Based on this initial configuration, alternative processes exploiting the continuous simulated countercurrent approach have been specifically developed and investigated for both capture and polishing of biologics. The main advantages brought by these techniques with respect to batch, single-column operations consist of: higher capacity utilization of the resin, higher productivity, lower buffer consumption and smaller environmental footprint (Lin et al., 2021). For what concerns the batch operation, there are many optimizations that can be pursued in terms of operating parameter adjustment in order to improve the performances. The loadings can be decreased, as well as the gradient slope, to improve the peak separations and consequently the final purity in the product elution window (PEW). In this way, the PEW boundaries can be modified considering a bigger width, so as to increase the target product yield. Nevertheless, these actions negatively affect the specific solvent consumption and the productivity of the process, as a consequence of the lower amount of material loaded onto the column.

Another option to improve the process performance is to change the resin, going towards smaller particle size. Indeed, most of the chromatographic processes are diffusion-limited: the diffusion of the molecules inside and outside the particles takes place with a much lower rate with respect to the convective flow in the mobile phase, which is driven by the applied buffer flow rates. This significantly impacts the final selectivity between the species at the column outlet and, as a consequence, the purity drops down. This negative phenomenon can be tackled by exploiting smaller particle size, so as to decrease the distance for the molecules to be travelled in the stationary phase: in this way the broadness of the different peaks is narrowed down, leading to a higher final target product purity. Nonetheless, considering lower particle size, the backpressure inside the column increases and lower flow rates have to be used, decreasing the productivity of the process (Chibério et al., 2020; De Luca et al., 2020; Steinebach et al., 2017; Vogg et al., 2019).

These limitations can be overcome exploiting continuous countercurrent techniques with multi-column operation units, in which the purity specification can be satisfied increasing at the same time the final yield. This improved performance comes as a consequence of the interconnected steps between two columns that are present in all the different technologies already developed. With this novel approach, the portions of the chromatogram in which the purity is not satisfied are automatically captured in the downstream column for further processing. This allows to keep the yield high in the polishing step, and to maximize the resin utilization in the capture step.

The main limitation relative to a continuous countercurrent process following the SMB approach is related to the possibility of handling binary mixtures only. The impurities that need to be removed with these processes should behave similarly, so that they can be safely lumped up in a single pseudo compound. It is also worth mentioning the complexity of the experimental setup, in which the experiments could involve up to 16 columns (Chen et al., 2021). This of course increases the likeliness of a failure of the many valves involved in the operation, but it also represents a problem for the backpressure that can be generated during the interconnected phases of the process. This would force the operator to decrease the flow rates, negatively impacting the final productivity and the specific buffer consumption of the process. Nowadays, this problem has been already minimized, as few continuous chromatographic technologies implementing the countercurrent principle with only two to three columns have been developed, as it is for the multi-column countercurrent solvent gradient purification (MCSGP) technique used for the polishing step (Aumann and Morbidelli, 2008; Baur et al., 2016; Bigelow et al., 2021; Jungbauer, 2013; Kim et al., 2021; Krättli et al., 2013; Müller-Späth et al., 2013a; Nicoud, 2014; Steinebach et al., 2016; Ströhlein et al., 2006; Ulmer et al., 2017; Vogg et al., 2020).

Another potential drawback to be considered is the non-linearity of the adsorption equilibria of the different compounds present in the crude that, due to the accumulations of the species inside the system, can shift their retention times cycle by cycle. This is a huge problem undermining the process robustness, as the steady state condition may not be reached affecting the final performances in terms of the predicted outputs. It is the main reason why most of the companies, nowadays, adopt batch, single-column experiment-based approaches to optimize at most the prediction of the continuous, multi-column experiments. Most of the times this turns out to be inefficient and time consuming and one possible solution to the problem that is gaining more and more interest is the development of mechanistic models for the description of the process. This would represent a huge improvement in terms of efficiency of the process, prediction of peak evolutions over time, buffer consumption and overall productivity of the operation (Chen et al., 2021; Lin et al., 2021). It is still to be mentioned that for such an approach, the isotherm parameters are required for all of the species in the system. This can be labor intensive as it typically requires the development of regression or fitting algorithms to determine these parameters from specifically designed experiments.

In the following section, we focus the attention on the continuous countercurrent technologies currently available for the purification ofbiologics and based on frontal chromatography. The countercurrent processes that are based on the bind and elute approach are covered in chapter "Application of Multicolumn Countercurrent Solvent Gradient Purification to the polishing of therapeutic proteins" by Catani and De Luca, instead. For each of the processes investigated, we will deepen the working principles and go through some examples of purifications successfully completed, in order to highlight the advantages that these processes bring about compared to their batch, single-column counterparts.

## 3. Continuous countercurrent frontal chromatographic technologies

### 3.1 CaptureSMB

Frontal chromatography is mainly implemented for the capture step, with the aim of separating the product from process-related impurities. Used mainly for the purification of monoclonal antibodies (mAbs) and Fc-fusion proteins, the process should aim at obtaining product pools with high yield and throughput as well as a concentration of the product, important for the volume compression of the subsequent unit operations (Angarita et al., 2015; Follman and Fahrner, 2004; Ghose et al., 2005; Hahn, 2003; Shukla et al., 2007). A relevant parameter that has to be considered for these types of processes is the dynamic binding capacity (DBC) of the resin, whose value, which is a function of the residence time, expresses the amount of material that can be loaded onto the column until a certain percentage of the feed concentration is reached in the eluate. A reference value for the acceptable breakthrough in the capture step is 1% of the feed concentration, which avoids wasting to much valuable product. The $DBC_{1\%BT}$ can be calculated according to Eq. (1):

$$DBC_{1\%BT}\ (g/L) = \frac{EV_{1\%} \times C_{feed}}{CV} \tag{1}$$

where $C_{feed}$ is the initial crude concentration, $EV_{1\%}$ the elution volume when 1% of the feed concentration is measured in the eluate from the column and CV is the column volume. As such, the $DBC_{1\%BT}$ is often considered to determine the maximum loading duration in a single-column frontal operation. The proper design of the process therefore relies on the accurate measurement of the DBC from breakthrough experiments. In Fig. 4, a typical breakthrough curve (BTC) is shown. Its shape largely

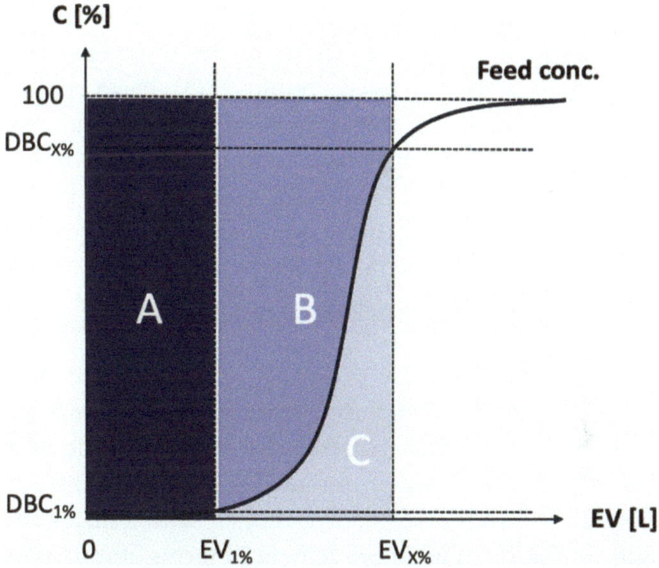


**Fig. 4** Illustration of a breakthrough curve (BTC) represented as product concentration at the column outlet (C) (expressed as a percentage of the feed concentration) vs. elution volume (EV). $EV_{1\%}$ and $EV_{X\%}$ are the elution volumes corresponding to an outlet concentration of respectively 1% ($DBC_{1\%}$) and X% ($DBC_{X\%}$) of the feed concentration. The portion A is related to the batch capacity utilization, while A+B is the capacity utilization achievable with a CaptureSMB process.

depends on the thermodynamics of the resin-protein interactions and the mass-transfer limitations in the pores of the resin. In the case of instantaneous mass transfer in the solid phase, the breakthrough curve would look like a step, corresponding to a loaded volume equal to the equilibrium binding capacity of the resin. The deviation from this ideal behavior, leading to the typical sigmoidal BTC, is introduced by mass-transfer limitations in the pores as well as by radial diffusion. As mentioned above, it is common for a single-column operation to work close to the $DBC_{1\%}$, often adopting an 80–90% safety margin. This is mainly done to avoid product losses, elongate the column lifetime in terms of resin capacity, due to aggressive cleaning causing ligand leaching, but also to obtain consistent data, avoiding some possible variabilities due to different resin-ligand density and column packing (Angarita et al., 2015). This situation is sketched by the region A in Fig. 2, which is associated to a very poor column loading and hence poor column utilization. This is a tremendous limitation, in particular for Protein A affinity resins, whose cost is about one order of magnitude higher than a non-affinity one. This brings also to a huge loss in terms of specific buffer consumption, since an unnecessary amount of solvent is used to clean the portion of the column remained unutilized (Mahajan et al., 2012).

The need for maximizing the capacity utilization, and reducing the buffer, in order to maximize the cost savings inspired the development of the CaptureSMB process from YMC ChromaCon. This is a continuous twin-column technology based on the simulated countercurrent configuration that was initially thought for the Protein A affinity chromatography, but that with minimal modifications can be extended to other chromatographic purifications.

The flow diagram of a single cycle of CaptureSMB is schematized in Fig. 5. The idea behind this technology is to use two columns, alternatively operated in batch or interconnected, in order to allow the downstream column to capture the breakthrough from the upstream one. This in fact allows safely loading the columns up to their $DBC_{70\%}$, with a major advantage in terms of resin utilization. The improvement in terms of capacity utilization can be appreciated from Fig. 4, in which a general BTC is represented. While in a single-column operation the product loaded to the column is only represented by the area of the region A, in a CaptureSMB this amount can be pushed to include also the region B. In fact, the product lost in the breakthrough from the upstream column, represented by the area of region C, can be captured by the downstream column that is interconnected through a system of valves.

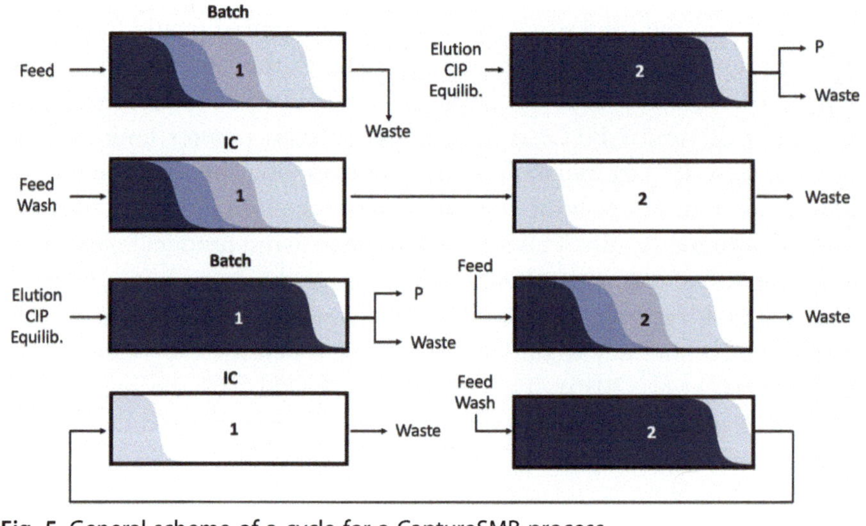


**Fig. 5** General scheme of a cycle for a CaptureSMB process.

Then, one cycle can be divided in two symmetric switches, in which the columns are sequentially connected, *i.e.*, interconnected (IC) phase, and disconnected, *i.e.*, batch phase, and eventually are exchanged in position at the end of each switch. The cycle is completed when both columns passed through four different operations: loading, washing, elution and regeneration.

Following the scheme of Fig. 5, in the first batch phase, the column 1 is fed with the outlet line connected to the waste stream. Usually, the loading is provided up to the above-mentioned batch safety limit, in order not to waste the product, so as the 80-90% of $DBC_{1\%}$. At the same time, in the column 2 the product elution and the consequent collection is performed. During a typical CaptureSMB run, prior to start the elution, the salt concentration inside the column is increased to throw all the remaining species bound to the resin through non-specific interactions during the previous cycles. Then, the salt concentration and the pH are decreased with the proper elution buffer to collect the product attached to the stationary phase. After the elution, the column 2 is cleaned, regenerated and equilibrated while it is connected to the waste stream. The first batch is usually performed with a low loading flow rate, in order to increase the $DBC_{1\%}$ for the fed column 1. On the other hand, the flow rates of the regeneration phase for column 2 is higher, in order to match the time.

As soon as the safety limit for the batch loading of the column 1 is reached, the column 1 and 2 are interconnected. Then, in the first IC step, the column 1 is fed until a $DBC_{x\%}$, where the X% is usually a value between 60% and 70%, depending on the shape of the BTC. Subsequently, the breakthrough is collected by the downstream column 2 (region C in Fig. 4) and once the $DBC_{x\%}$ is reached, the column 1 is washed to let the unbound material to be kept by the downstream column. Once this step is finished, the first switch is completed and the same operations are repeated exchanging the column positions, by switching the valves to properly set the flow paths.

It is worth mentioning that, except for the feeding of the column in the batch phase, for all the other steps, *i.e.*, the elution and regeneration batch steps and the IC ones, the flow rates can be increased as much as possible, so as to maximize the overall productivity and the specific buffer consumption of the process.

Moreover, a startup procedure is initially required, in which a prolonged sequential loading is used, to reach the steady state condition from the second cycle.

As reported in detail in the work by Angarita et al. (2015), there are different operating parameters to be set and their determination requires a certain procedure to be followed. In the batch phase, the operating parameters are the feed flow rate ($Q_B$) and the relative duration ($t_B$). Similarly, the IC phase includes the feed flow rate ($Q_{IC}$), the feeding duration ($t_{IC}$), the washing flow rate ($Q_{IC,wash}$) and its corresponding duration ($t_{IC,wash}$).

The optimal operating parameters of the CaptureSMB are determined from the BTC obtained with single-column, batch experiments. At first, three BTCs are considered: two at the desired $Q_{IC}$, with one column (1C) and two columns (2C) in series, and the third one is recorded with 1C and a lower flow rate, typically equal to 50% of $Q_{IC}$ ($Q_L$). From these BTCs some EVs are obtained:

- $EV_{QIC,1\%,1C}$: elution volume related to the 1% outlet feed concentration ($DBC_{1\%}$), using a single column and the desired IC feeding flow rate $Q_{IC}$.
- $EV_{QIC,X\%,1C}$: elution volume related to the X% outlet feed concentration ($DBC_{X\%}$) (where X% is a value between 60% and 70% as mentioned before), using a single column and the desired IC feeding flow rate $Q_{IC}$.
- $EV_{QIC,1\%,2C}$: elution volume related to the 1% outlet feed concentration ($DBC_{1\%}$), with two columns in series, using the desired IC feeding flow rate $Q_{IC}$.
- $EV_{QL,1\%,1C}$: elution volume related to the 1% outlet feed concentration ($DBC_{1\%}$), using a single column and the lower flow rate $Q_L$.
- $EV_y$: elution volume equal to the smallest one between $EV_{QIC,X\%,1C}$ and $EV_{QIC,1\%,2C}$. Usually the biggest one is $EV_{QIC,1\%,2C}$, unless the process is characterized by very shallow BTCs.

During the IC step, the feed breaking through the upstream column can be considered as a pre-load (PL), which can be calculated according to Eq. (2).

$$PL\ (g/L) = \frac{Area_{EV_y} \times C_{feed}}{CV} \tag{2}$$

where $Area_{EVy}$ is the integral of the BTC up to $EV_y$, $C_{feed}$ is the initial crude concentration in g/L and CV is the column volume in L. In Fig. 4, PL is related to the portion C of the plot. The downstream pre-loaded column then, during the following switch in the batch operation, is fed up to a certain target loading (TL), calculated as in Eq. (3).

$$TL\ (g/L) = \frac{\left(Z\% \times EV_{QL,1\%,1C} - V_{dead}\right) \times C_{feed}}{CV} - PL \tag{3}$$

where $V_{dead}$ is the dead volume of the column and Z% a safety margin, usually set to 80%, to consider the column degradation over time. The mentioned start-up procedure, with the loading provided up to the PL of the downstream column to reach the steady state from the second cycle, has a duration ($t_{start\text{-}up}$) that is calculated according to Eq. (4).

$$t_{start-up}\ (min) = \frac{EV_y - V_{dead}}{Q_{IC}} \tag{4}$$

The feeding flow rate used during the batch configuration is then calculated as in Eq. (5).

$$Q_B\ (L/\ min) = \frac{TL \times CV}{C_{feed} \times t_B} \tag{5}$$

where $t_B$ represents the duration of the batch phase. The duration of the IC step ($t_{IC}$) can be calculated according to Eq. (6).

$$t_{IC}\ (min) = \frac{EV_y - Z\% \times EV_{QL,1\%,1C} + \left(\frac{TL \times CV}{C_{feed}}\right) - Q_B \times t_B}{Q_{IC}} \tag{6}$$

The evaluation of the process performance of a CaptureSMB process is done by comparison with respect to some batch, single-column experiments. The process performance parameters to quantify the relative improvement of the results can be related to the product quality of the collected fraction (in %). In addition to this output, the final target product concentration (g/L) and the amount of impurities present in the final pool can be considered. Usually, the last one is referred in percentage for aggregates and in parts per million (ppm) for smaller impurities and fragments as the host-cell proteins (HCPs) and the DNA. The overall performance can be also established in terms of yield (%) of the target product, considering the total mass of product collected with respect to the initial amount fed onto the column, and the load per cycle (g/L) that quantifies the capacity utilization of the resin. Other performance parameters usually considered are the productivity (g/L/h), that is related to the amount of recovered product per column volume per total process duration, and the specific buffer consumption (L/g) that refers to the total volume of the consumed buffer per gram of purified product.

The improvements brought by the CaptureSMB with respect to batch is already well established and many works are available in literature.

In Müller-Späth et al. (2013b) the CaptureSMB was implemented for the purification of a monoclonal antibody (mAb), the IgG1, from clarified cell culture harvest using the Amsphere JWT 203 Protein A stationary phase. In this work, for constant productivity and recovery, the capacity utilization was improved from 40% to 90% with the load per cycle that increased from 16.3 g/L, corresponding to the $DBC_{1\%}$ of the batch run, to 36.5 g/L. The target product concentration in the pool increases by 1023%, from 3.3 to 7.3 g/L, which is important for the compression of the following unit operations and at the same time the specific buffer consumption of the process decreased by 45%.

In Müller-Späth et al. (2013c) the CaptureSMB was carried out always considering a monoclonal antibody IgG1 as a case study, using Amsphere JWT 203 protein A stationary phase. In this case the comparison between CaptureSMB and batch was done considering different maximum feed flow rates, from 150 to 600 cm/h. For similar amount of impurities in the final product pool, it was detected a higher yield of the CaptureSMB with respect to batch: while the yield ranges from 87% to 93% in the batch for the different tested linear flow rates, for the CaptureSMB this range increases to 87–95%. Moreover, the productivity increases for the continuous process for all the linear flow rates, with a maximum improvement of 35% at 600 cm/h. While the buffer consumption remains almost constant in the two processes, the load per cycle increases for all the linear flow rates: this is mainly due to the fact that in the CaptureSMB this output is less dependent from the feed flow rate since the load of the column to be eluted is maximized through the sequential loading phase.

In Ulmer et al. (2015), a purification of mAb fragments, previously produced by the digestion of IgGs present in a clarified cell culture harvest, was performed with the CaptureSMB using YMC Japan ECOplus AB self-packed columns filled with Cytiva Capto L resin. Also in this case, an overall improvement of the performance was obtained with respect to batch: the yield increases from 80% to 105%, as well as the concentration of the target product in the pool, that increases from 1.4 to 3.1 g/L. The load per cycle increased as it happened for the previous cases, from 9.2 to 15.0 g/L. The productivity increased by 93% and the specific buffer consumption decreased by 54%. In this work, an interesting economic evaluation was done: this analysis shows that considering the resin costs of the Capto L, performing the CaptureSMB instead of a batch, single-column capture process, the costs decrease from 5 million dollars to 3 million dollars per year, with an overall cost saving of more than 30%.

Overall, the CaptureSMB process demonstrated very effective in increasing the resin utilization, alleviating the yield-resin utilization tradeoff typically in place for single-column operations. This is particularly relevant when applied to the Protein A affinity chromatography, whose cost of goods are largely covered by the cost of the resin itself. Hence, increasing the utilization of the resin means an important improvement in terms of process sustainability.

## 3.2 Flow2

Despite the frontal chromatography is widely spread in the biopharmaceutical market for the capture process, this technology is gaining interest as an alternative to the bind and elute processes also for particular polishing operations, due to its high productivity and simple experimental setup implementation. It is the case for example of the removal of mAb aggregates from the product. Aggregation may in fact occur in the eluate from the Protein A capture, due to the acidic pH used for elution, so that an efficient polishing with high throughput is required for the elimination of such high molecular weight impurities that can introduce immunogenicity concerns. With respect to a typical frontal Protein A affinity chromatography, in which the product is first adsorbed and then eluted after the impurity removal, as described in the previous Section, for the polishing step the usual way to proceed is the opposite. A proper resin, an ion-exchange one in most cases, is selected to adsorb the impurities, while letting the product flowing through the column without being adsorbed.

Then, in a typical flow-through (FT) process using an ion-exchanger, the aggregates are retained in the stationary phase and the product flows through with the mobile phase. Moreover, a displacement effect might take place inside the column, for which the target component bound to the resin is pushed out by the more strongly adsorbed aggregates, resulting in a higher concentration of the target component in the product pool than in the crude material (Carta and Jungbauer, 2010; Reck et al., 2017; Vogg et al., 2020).

A batch, single-column implementation for this process consists of three consecutive steps. In the first phase, the column, pre-equilibrated with the proper buffers, is fed with the crude material. During this step, the target component breaking through the column is collected. This stage can be continued until the impurities start breaking through as well, progressively reducing the purity of the product pool as the loading is protracted. Therefore, as soon as a minimum acceptable purity is reached, the feeding is interrupted and a washing step is performed to collect the remaining product in the voids and interstices or loosely bound to the stationary phase. The maximum feed loading volume is then limited to small values of breakthrough (*i.e.*, 3–5%) of the impurities. Finally, in the last step, the column regeneration takes place with strip, cleaning-in-place (CIP) and re-equilibration. In batch mode, the operating parameters to be optimized are then the flow rates and the relative durations of each step, as well as the modifier concentration during the wash.

The parameters that are considered for evaluating the process performance are the purity (%), given typically as a constraint, the product yield (%) of the final collected fraction and the overall productivity (g/L/h) of the process.

In this type of process, the critical phase is represented by the wash. During the loading, the collected product is characterized by a very high purity that usually meets the specific biomanufacturing requirements. Then, while the wash is performed in order to increase the total product recovery, the weakly bound impurities start co-eluting contaminating the final purity. The longer this washing phase and the higher the product recovery, but at the same time the lower the purity, because of more and more impurities collected in the product pool. It results that a single-column batch frontal chromatography is affected by a limiting purity-yield tradeoff.

In this perspective, a FT continuous countercurrent process for the polishing of mAbs from high molecular weight aggregates, namely the Flow2 process, was designed to tackle the limitations of a batch process with a twin-column system (Shi et al., 2021a; Vogg et al., 2020).

A schematic illustration of one cycle of the Flow2 process is represented in Fig. 6, in which two identical columns are considered in terms of dimension. One cycle is formed by two switches: in the first switch, column 1 is placed upstream of column 2, then during the second switch the columns exchange their positions, switching properly the valves of the system, so as to have the column 2 located upstream of column 1. Since the two switches are identical except for the column position, only the first switch is described in the following.

During the first inter-connected (IC) phase, the loading is performed with the two columns in series and the product flowing through the column 2 is collected at its outlet. In the second IC step of the first switch, the washing is performed to desorb all the target component still bound to the stationary phase in column 1. In the meanwhile, an inline dilution (ID) is applied between the two columns, to restore binding conditions prior to

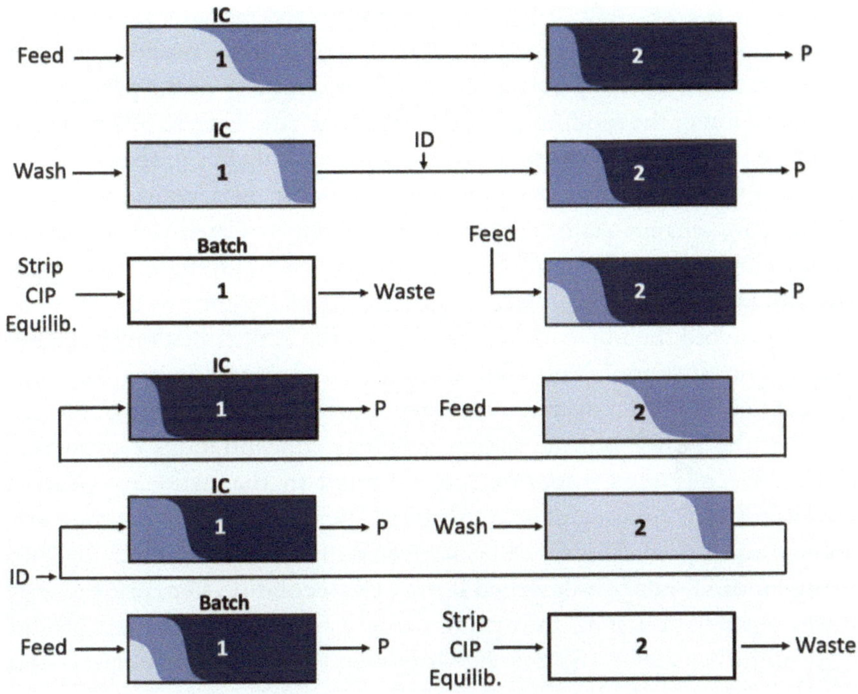


**Fig. 6** General scheme of a cyclic-steady state Flow2 process, where the target product is represented in dark blue and the lighter blues are related to the impurities.

enter in the downstream column. While the washing is performed, the product collection is still made at the outlet of the column 2. In the last batch phase, in which the columns are disconnected from each other, the column 1 is regenerated with strip, CIP and re-equilibration and the column 2 is loaded with fresh feed material. After this, as described before, the columns exchange their positions, and the second switch is done completing one cycle.

Looking into the outlet streams illustrated in Fig. 6, it is clear that throughout the entire duration of the process, the product is continuously collected at the outlet of the downstream column, while the loading is just interrupted during the washing step. As a consequence of this, the only phase in which there could be some product loss is the batch one, while the upstream column is regenerated.

In this Flow2 the operating parameters are manifold: the durations and the relative flow rates of each step, including also the one of the ID stream during the wash, the modifier concentrations during the wash and the ID factor.

The ID is a key step, to be carefully optimized, because it is source of improvement in terms of process performance, but if not properly designed can break down the final purity, yield and productivity of the process. The concentration of the modifier, as well as the flow rate, have to be set in order to restore the binding condition of the buffer resulting in a proper ID factor. The major improvement that this step can bring, in a typical process in which ion-exchange resins are involved, is mainly related to the fact that the washing step can be performed with higher ionic strength with respect to batch. During the single-column process, the wash buffer ionic strength is limited to avoid the impurity desorption and the contamination of the final collected product pool. This mild washing also compromises the amount of product that can be recovered in this step, thus limiting the yield of the process. For the Flow2 instead, higher modifier concentrations can be used, because the desorbed impurities are rebound to the stationary phase of the downstream column, after appropriate ID, without reducing the purity of the product pool. This results in an overall improvement of the final yield because more product is desorbed during the second IC step, prior to enter in the regeneration step, thus minimizing the above-mentioned product losses of the last step of the switch. Moreover, the productivity can be optimized maximizing the ID flow rate and, from this perspective, it is important to keep track of the total flow rate received by the downstream column, not bringing the pressure above the maximum limit sustainable by the resin and the column housing.

It is worth mentioning that before and after the Flow2 process, a start-up and a shutdown method are performed, respectively. In the start-up, the column 1 is loaded in batch mode, collecting the product at its outlet, and the feeding is similar to the one performed at the inlet of the downstream column in the Flow2 batch phase. This is done to favor the achievement of the steady state in the next cycles. The shutdown method is then performed after the last cycle in steady state: the loaded column in the batch phase of the last switch is washed, its outflow is collected as product and the regeneration lastly takes place. As it happens usually for any kind of continuous countercurrent processes, the start-up and the shutdown are not considered for the final calculations of the performance parameters.

In Vogg et al. (2020), the Flow2 process was designed to compare its design space and performance robustness with respect to a batch, single-column process. In this work, two identical columns Eshmuno CP-FT from Merck were used to purify a binary mixture composed by a monovalent monomer of 100 kDa and aggregates. The optimal operating parameters for the continuous process were set through a mathematical model and the results were compared with two different FT batch processes. The ID was demonstrated to have an important role in relaxing the constraints on the washing buffer composition, whose ionic strength can be increased to desorb and improve the yield. Moreover, despite the productivity between the multi-column and the batch processes is the same, it was found that the Flow2 allows to maintain a larger design space with constant performance related to some operating parameter perturbations, so that the process was more robust exploiting the continuous countercurrent mode of operation.

Similarly, Shi et al. (2021a) developed an *ad-hoc* design procedure for the simulation and optimization of the Flow2 process and compared its performance with a batch process for the purification of a general mixture of mAbs and the corresponding high molecular weight (HMW) impurities. Exploiting a chromatographic lumped kinetic approach with linear driving force approximation, it was shown that, considering optimal operating conditions for both batch and Flow2, the latter allowed to alleviate the yield-productivity tradeoff when a minimum tolerable purity was set. In particular, with the Flow2 it was possible to access higher productivities than the batch at comparable process yield. Moreover, the robustness was demonstrated to be higher for the Flow2 process considering the perturbation of several operating parameters: loading flow rate, washing buffer ionic strength and loading duration. This was mainly attributed to the stabilization operated by the inline dilution, which could not only improve the performances of the process through an improved product recovery, but also compensated the perturbations of the main operating parameters.

Overall, the Flow2 process was demonstrated a valid option for the purification of mAbs from their aggregates, with high purity, throughput and process robustness.

## 3.3 BioSMB

BioSMB from Sartorius is an alternative continuous multi-column countercurrent operation allowing key benefits in the capture step. In application, the BioSMB relies on the adsorption of the product breaking through the upstream column in the downstream one, during an interconnected loading operation (Ayturk, 2015; Bisschops, 2012, 2015; Gjoka et al., 2015; Najera, 2016; Ötes et al., 2018; Utturkar et al., 2019a). Enhanced process economics by improvement of the productivity and resin utilization are also highlighted in process development using BioSMB (Bisschops, 2015; Najera, 2016;

Ötes et al., 2018). In addition to the advantages, it allows for single-use manufacturing as its valves that direct the flow paths to and from all columns are designed in a disposable cassette (Bisschops, 2012). Therefore, if the BioSMB system is configured with single-use columns and membranes or other single-use chromatographic devices, the process becomes a single-use chromatography (Bisschops, 2012). This peculiarity is introduced to address the need for more sterile, contaminant-free environments, which is leading to the rise of the demand for single-use systems. This is of paramount importance especially in the production of vaccines and biologics. In the single-use system, the reduction of cleaning steps by avoiding cleaning validation processes and ensuring robust product profiles by removing variabilities in column packing are offered that appeal to industrial applications (Bisschops, 2012; Utturkar et al., 2019a).

As typical for these systems, the optimization of a BioSMB process requires the accurate determination of the dynamic binding capacity of the resin under different conditions. Therefore, breakthrough experiments are performed at varying residence times and feed concentrations. The columns are overloaded until the product concentration at the outlet of column 1 ($C_{out,1}$) reaches 90–100% of the initial concentration of the target ($C_0$), as shown in Fig. 7A and B, where $t_{DBC}$ is the time point when the product breaks through the outlet of the column in series. In Fig. 7B, the two BTCs of the product are depicted, which are detected by two different UV sensors. At the outlet of each sensor, the breakthrough of the columns is detected, and in the case of the first column, the breakthrough target enters the second column; in the case of the second column, the breakthrough of the target is discarded. The different adsorption amounts of the target are labelled as X and Y. To calculate the optimal operating binding capacity (OBC), a number of columns ($N_{Col}$) is taken into consideration in operating BioSMB to obtain the BTC of the first column and the last column in series (Gjoka et al., 2015). In case of $N_{Col}=2$, in which the two columns are connected in series, each column has a residence time of $\theta$, and thus $2\theta$ will be the total residence time for the two columns. In this calculation, the shape of the BTC is assumed to be shifted only by the residence time. This means that the BTC of the two columns in series, each with a residence time of $\theta$, will have the same shape of the BTC of a single column with $2\theta$. Therefore, instead of testing the columns in series, changing of the retention time, or $\theta$, to simulate the BTCs for any number of columns can be conducted. For example, to test the fifth column as the last column in series, $5\theta$ is used as the residence time instead of $\theta$. This provides the BTC of the fifth column, using only one column (Gjoka et al., 2015).

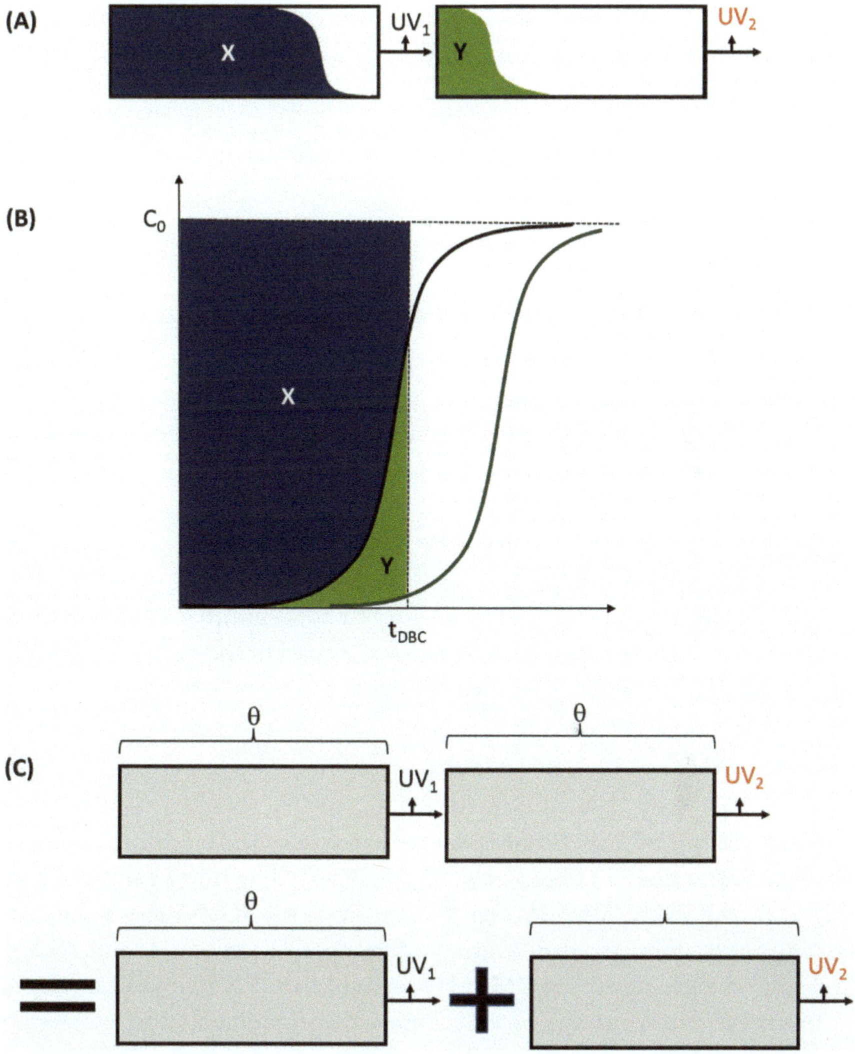


**Fig. 7** (A) Two interconnected columns in series under breakthrough conditions. (B) A breakthrough test using the two columns in series. In the breakthrough, adsorption of X and Y amount of the target on the first column and second column, respectively. The black and orange lines represent the breakthrough of the first column and second column, respectively. (C) Experimental design of breakthrough tests for the first and last column by varying retention times.

Using Eq. (6), the ideal OBC, which is the amount of product adsorbed immediately before the breakthrough of the first column, can be obtained.

$$OBC = \int_{0}^{Q \times t_{DBC}} \frac{[C_0 - C_{out,1}]dv}{CV} \tag{7}$$

The time for a cycle ($t_c$) can be calculated following Eq. (8).

$$t_c = t_L \times N_L + t_R + t_I \tag{8}$$

in which $N_L$ is the number of columns in the load feed, $t_R$ is the "rest" time that is the wash, elution, regeneration, and equilibration phases, and $t_I$ is the idle time, which is a time interval between the end of equilibration and start of load, $t_L$ is the load time derived from the OBC in Eq. (9):

$$t_L = OBC \times \frac{\theta}{C_0} \tag{9}$$

$N_{Col}$ is obtained using Eq. (10) to decide the total number of the columns required to operate the BioSMB. When the sum of $t_L$ and $t_R$ is not divisible, $t_I$ is introduced to obtain a whole number.

$$N_{Col} = roundup\left(\frac{t_L \times N_L + t_R}{t_L}\right) \tag{10}$$

Implementation of the BioSMB system to two mAb chromatography processes is described in Gjoka et al. (2015, 2017). The unit operations considered in the study were Protein A capture using KANEKA KanCapA, flow-through anion exchange using Mustang Q membrane, and mixed-mode cation exchange using CMM HyperCel MMCEX (Gjoka et al., 2015).

In the Protein A capture process, before the implementation, a design of experiment (DoE) was performed to optimize overloading, wash volume, feed concentration, and residence time. In the design space of the continuous mode, more than 50% of increased OBC and an increased linear flow rate for the load feed were found (Gjoka et al., 2017). The linear flow rate in the design space was 720 cm/h, which exceeded the recommended maximum linear velocity of the Protein A column (500 cm/h), In this case, the flow was split in two pairs of the columns in series, having four columns at the load feed at any given point (Gjoka et al., 2017). The idle time was minimized by introducing four additional columns for each phase, which was wash, elution, CIP, and re-equilibration as shown in Fig. 8 (Gjoka et al., 2017).

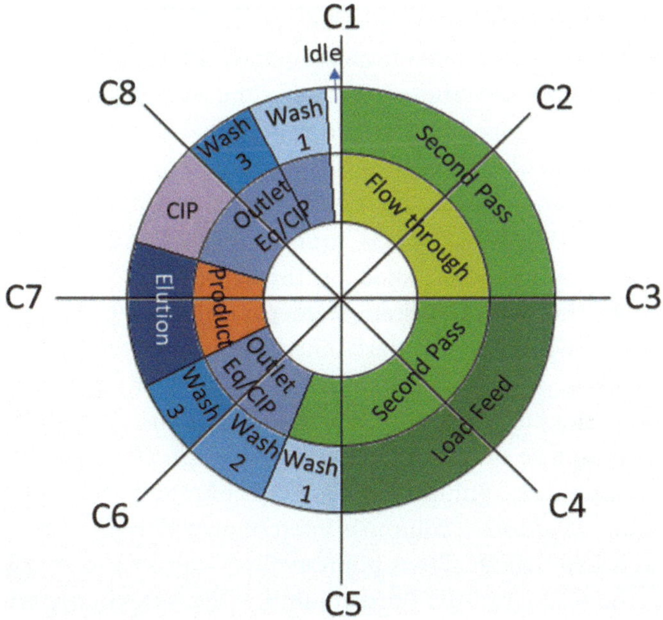


**Fig. 8** Chronogram of the Protein A Chromatography in the BioSMB system. The eight columns for the process are shown as radial spokes. The outer and inner rings represent input and output of the columns. The cycle is run in clockwise direction.

In processing 25 L of harvested cell culture fluid, 284% productivity improvement and 96% resin volume reduction compared to its batch process (Gjoka et al., 2017).

The polishing steps of anion exchange and cation exchange chromatography were designed in flow-through mode for the removal of HCP and aggregates. Investigation of different conductivity and pH load conditions for the removal of the impurities was performed by a DoE to find an optimal load condition (Gjoka et al., 2015). Using the optimal condition, the reduction of the resin volume by 74% was achieved with comparable impurity removal compared to its batch process in the anion exchange process (Gjoka et al., 2017). Further removal of HCP and mAb aggregates was completed with the cation exchange process. Investigation of trade-off between the impurity removal and OBC was performed by running a column-based DoE using different pH (Gjoka et al., 2017). The optimal operational condition successfully reduced the resin volume by 97% compared to its batch process. Moreover, the overall buffer consumption in the continuous processes was reduced by 44% compared to the batch processes (Gjoka et al., 2017).

## 3.4 Periodic countercurrent chromatography

In the periodic countercurrent chromatography (PCC), three or more chromatography columns are employed to offer the advantages of SMB, which are the productivity gain by increased resin utilization and cost savings by reduced buffer and column footprints compared to the single-column operations (Godawat et al., 2012; Gomis-Fons et al., 2020; Shi et al., 2021b; Utturkar et al., 2019b). ÄKTA PCC from Cytiva is considered the standard in this field, with a process based on three (3C-PCC) or four columns (4C-PCC). In the 3-PCC system, two parallel flow paths are featured. One involving two columns interconnected in series and the second one for the remaining column operated in batch. In a first stage, the interconnection is exploited to overload the upstream column, allowing the downstream one to capture the product breaking through. The second flow path allows cleaning and re-equilibrating the third column. In the second stage of the process, the overloaded column is interconnected to the regenerated one for a washing step, which allows improved recovery of the product. At the same time, the feeding of the third column, which previously received the breakthrough is continued in batch. The columns are periodically exchanged in position until everyone has acted in each of the three roles. It results that a 3C-PCC cycle is composed by 6 stages, as shown in Fig. 9 (Godawat et al., 2012; Gomis-Fons et al., 2020). The 4C-PCC applies the same principle but is more advantageous for its use when the 3C-PCC system has a rate limiting step in the regeneration and re-equilibration (RR) step (Godawat et al., 2012; Shi et al., 2021b). By addition of an additional flow path for the fourth column, the RR step can be split into two and thus becomes no longer the rate limiting step (Godawat et al., 2012; Shi et al., 2021b). While CaptureSMB is operated in different feed flow rates for disconnected and interconnected modes, which are adjusted to be optimized as shown in Section 3.1, the BioSMB and PCC systems are operated at the same flow rate in the load feed and controlled by the predefined breakthrough level in the interconnected mode (Baur et al., 2016; Steinebach et al., 2016).

Various residence times for the interconnected load feed ($RT_C$), its corresponding load feed time in the interconnected mode ($t_C$), and different initial load feed concentrations ($C_0$) are tested for breakthrough experiments (Shi et al., 2021b). Using the data obtained from the breakthrough tests, breakthrough percentage of the first column(s) can be determined, which also affects $t_C$. Other time parameters that include the time for the RR

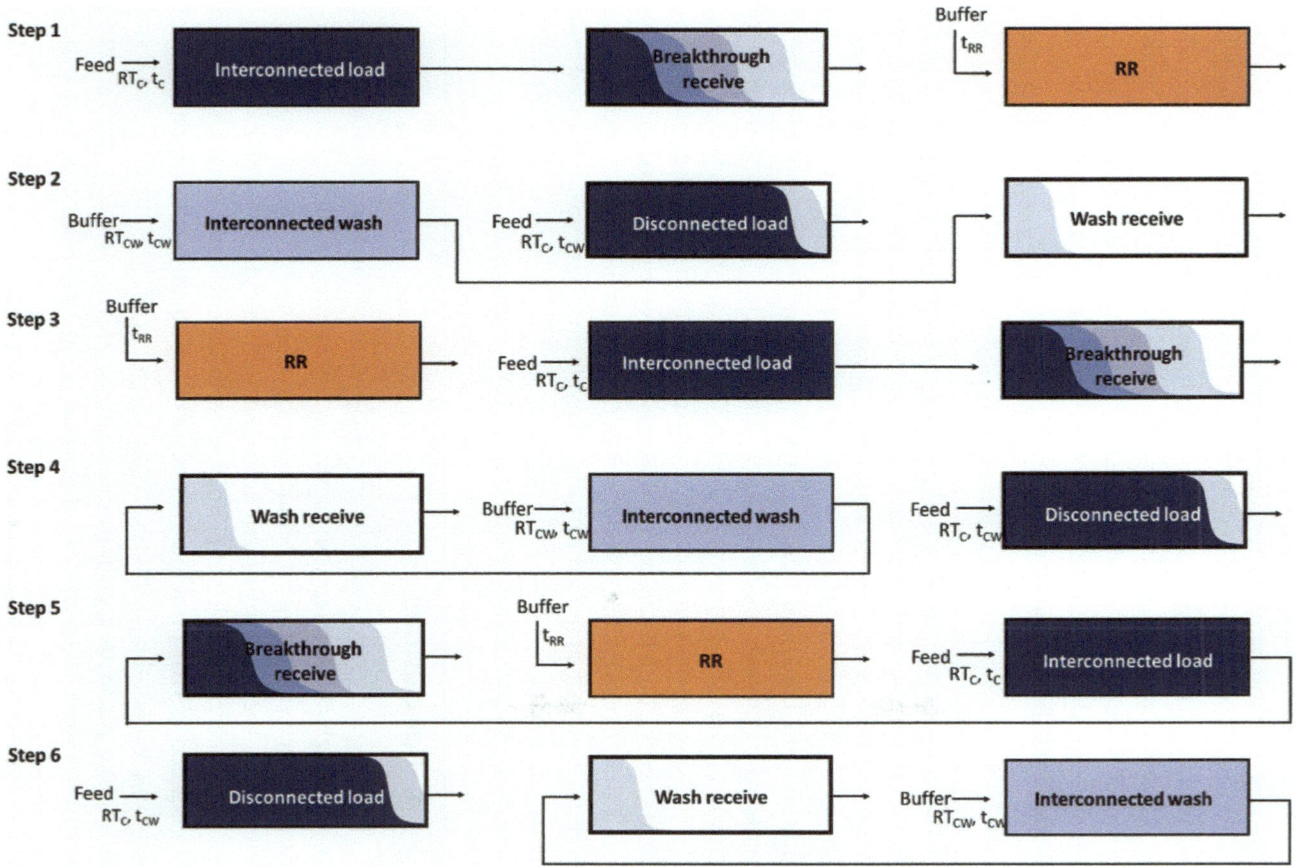


**Fig. 9** Schematic diagram of 3C-PCC.

step ($t_{RR}$), residence time for the interconnected wash ($RT_{CW}$), and its corresponding wash time in the interconnected mode ($t_{CW}$), are determined from one-column batch experiments (Shi et al., 2021b).

To obtain the lowest cycle time $t_{cycle}$, in the disconnected load feed, the load feed time is set to the wash time in the interconnected mode $t_{CW}$; and in the interconnected mode, the feed load time $t_C$ is set to be equal to the time for the RR step $t_{RR}$ (Shi et al., 2021b). When $t_C$ is not equal to $t_{RR}$, its difference needs to be introduced in the time for a cycle $t_{cycle}$ as the idle time in the BioSMB, defined as $t_{wait}$.

$$t_{wait} = 3|t_C - t_{RR}| \tag{11}$$

A case study of optimizing two objectives, increasing productivity and resin utilization compared to the batch operation, in the 3C-PCC system was conducted by Gomis-Fons et al. (2020). With the BTC data of Protein A column, process modeling using a general rate model (GRM) with parallel diffusion and Langmuir adsorption isotherm and multi-response experiments with varying residence times and load feed concentrations were applied in the two-objective 3C-PCC optimization (Gomis-Fons et al., 2020). Using the process parameters obtained from the modeling and experimental works, both batch and continuous mode were optimized for comparison. Pareto fronts for the comparison of the optimal batch to the continuous mode showed that, at the same productivity, from 30% to 75% enhanced resin utilization and, at the same resin utilization, from 70% to more than 200% improved productivity were obtained (Gomis-Fons et al., 2020).

## 4. Conclusions

In recent years, different multi-column continuous countercurrent flow-through chromatographic operations are being developed in the literature, to face the stringent regulations on biopharmaceuticals and, at the same time, the limitations encountered with single-column batch processes. Almost the whole panel of these techniques is based on the simulated moving bed (SMB) principle. It consists in simulating, through a series of switching valves, the countercurrent movement of the stationary phase and the mobile phase in a continuous fashion, so as to exploit the resulting enhanced mass transfer of the solutes to improve the separation performances.

These technologies are mainly developed for the capture step, allowing the removal of the so-called process-related impurities with high throughput and product recovery. In fact, they are specifically designed for the separation of binary mixtures. Hence, they are applicable to those cases where the impurities, although manifold, can be reasonably lumped up in a single pseudo component, with a homogeneous behavior with respect to the product. This indeed applies also to the removal of high molecular weight aggregates from the monomer, in particular in the case of mAbs after the acidification experienced during the Protein A affinity chromatography. Although an example of polishing step, a continuous flow-through process, namely the Flow2, has been proposed to overcome the limitations of the batch process. Distinctive feature of this process is its robustness to changes in key operating parameters, which makes it an ideal candidate for this operation.

On the other hand, for other polishing operations, which many times deal with central-cut separations, the preferred chromatographic mode is the bind and elute.

For the Protein A capture, three multi-column countercurrent flow-through processes have been developed and are discussed in this chapter, namely the CaptureSMB, BioSMB and 3C-PCC. For the accurate design of these processes, the measurement of the DBC through breakthrough experiments is an important prerequisite, as it regulates the duration of the loading in both batch and interconnected phases. The main outcome of these processes is an improvement of the resin utilization. Since the product breaking through the column can be captured in a second column interconnected in downstream position, the loading can be longer and hence the resin exploited more compared to a single-column process. This result is particularly relevant considering the high cost of a Protein A affinity resin, thus leading to an alleviation of the cost of goods associated to the process.

A crucial issue for a new biopharmaceutical process is the compliance with the current good manufacturing practices (cGMP), to reach regulatory approval and eventually scale-up to industrial settings. CaptureSMB, BioSMB, and PCC systems offered GMP complying case studies that satisfy not only cost effectiveness of the processes but also the regulatory aspects, while Flow2 was developed recently, and thus no industrial application was tested (Angelo et al., 2018; Mathiasson et al., 2020; Sartorius, 2021). High capital for installing a new production line, additional hardware investment, and, most importantly, regulatory aspects must be addressed as limiting factors in introducing the continuous chromatography systems. However, many case studies of successful implementation of the technology proved a concrete possibility to shift the focus of the downstream processing to these new applications.

## References

Andjelković U, Giacometti J, Josić D: Chapter 5—protein and peptide separations, In Fanali S, Haddad PR, Poole CF, Riekkola M-LBT-LC, editors: *Liquid chromatography*, ed 2, 2017, Elsevier, pp 107–157. https://doi.org/10.1016/B978-0-12-805392-8.00005-0.

Angarita M, et al.: Twin-column CaptureSMB: a novel cyclic process for protein A affinity chromatography, *J Chromatogr A* 1389:85–95, 2015.

Angelo J, et al.: Scale-up of twin-column periodic counter-current chromatography for MAb purification, *Bioprocess Int* 16, 2018.

Aumann L, Morbidelli M: A semicontinuous 3-column countercurrent solvent gradient purification (MCSGP) process, *Biotechnol Bioeng* 99:728–733, 2008.

Ayturk E: Leveraging large data sets in continuous chromatography applications: monitoring critical process parameters using MVDA capturing the value of continuous bioprocessing through MVDA, In Chetan Goudar, Amgen Inc. Suzanne Farid, Univ. Coll. London Christopher Hwang, Genzyme-Sanofi Karol Lacki, Novo Nord. Eds, ECI Symp. Ser. 2015.

Baur D, Angarita M, Müller-Späth T, Steinebach F, Morbidelli M: Comparison of batch and continuous multi-column protein A capture processes by optimal design, *Biotechnol J* 11:920–931, 2016.

Berruex, L. G. & Freitag, R. Separation and purification of biochemicals. in (ed. Meyers, R. A. B. T.-E. of Encyclopedia of physical science and technology ed 3, 651–673 (Academic Press, 2003). https://doi.org/10.1016/B0-12-227410-5/00683-9.

Bigelow E, et al.: Using continuous chromatography methodology to achieve high-productivity and high-purity enrichment of charge variants for analytical characterization, *J Chromatogr A* 1643, 2021, 462008.

Bisschops M: BioSMB$^{TM}$ technology: continuous countercurrent chromatography enabling a fully disposable process, *Biopharm Prod Technol* 1–2:769–791, 2012.

Bisschops M: BioSMB technology as an enabler for a fully continuous disposable biomanufacturing platform, *Contin Process Pharm Manuf*:35–52, 2015. https://doi.org/10.1002/9783527673681.ch02.

Broughton DB: Production-scale adsorptive separations of liquid mixtures by simulated moving-bed technology, *Sep Sci Technol* 19:723–736, 1984.

Broughton, D. B. & Gerhold, C. G. US Patent 2,985,589. (1961).

Carta G, Jungbauer A: Introduction to Protein Chromatography, *Protein Chromatography*:57–84, 2010. https://doi.org/10.1002/9783527630158.ch2.

Chen C-S, Konoike F, Yoshimoto N, Yamamoto S: A regressive approach to the design of continuous capture process with multi-column chromatography for monoclonal antibodies, *J Chromatogr A*, 2021. https://doi.org/10.1016/j.chroma.2021.462604, 462604.

Chibério, A. S. *et al.* Batch chromatography with recycle lag. II—Physical realization and experimental validation. J Chromatogr A **1623**, (2020).

Coskun O: Separation techniques: chromatography, *North Clin Istanbul* 3:156–160, 2016.

De la Torre BG, Albericio F: The pharmaceutical industry in 2017. An analysis of FDA Drug approvals from the perspective of molecules, *Molecules* 23, 2018.

De Luca C, et al.: Modern trends in downstream processing of biotherapeutics through continuous chromatography: the potential of multicolumn countercurrent solvent gradient purification, *TrAC - Trends Anal Chem* 132, 2020, 116051.

Follman DK, Fahrner RL: Factorial screening of antibody purification processes using three chromatography steps without protein A, *J Chromatogr A* 1024:79–85, 2004.

Freitag R: Displacement chromatography: application to downstream processing in biotechnology, *Bioseparation Bioprocess*:89–112, 1998. https://doi.org/10.1002/9783527619641.ch4.

Fritz JS: Early milestones in the development of ion-exchange chromatography: a personal account, *J Chromatogr A* 1039:3–12, 2004.

Ghose S, Allen M, Hubbard B, Brooks C, Cramer SM: Antibody variable region interactions with protein A: implications for the development of generic purification processes, *Biotechnol Bioeng* 92:665–673, 2005.

Gjoka X, Rogler K, Martino RA, Gantier R, Schofield M: A straightforward methodology for designing continuous monoclonal antibody capture multi-column chromatography processes, *J Chromatogr A* 1416:38–46, 2015.

Gjoka X, Gantier R, Schofield M: Transfer of a three step mAb chromatography process from batch to continuous: optimizing productivity to minimize consumable requirements, *J Biotechnol* 242:11–18, 2017.

Godawat R, et al.: Periodic countercurrent chromatography—design and operational considerations for integrated and continuous purification of proteins, *Biotechnol J* 7:1496–1508, 2012.

Gomis-Fons J, Andersson N, Nilsson B: Optimization study on periodic countercurrent chromatography integrated in a monoclonal antibody downstream process, *J Chromatogr A* 1621, 2020, 461055.

Hagel, L., Jagschies, G. & Sofer, G. 10—Optimization of chromatographic separations. in (eds. Hagel, L., Jagschies, G. & Sofer, G. B. T.-H. of Handbook of process chromatography ed 2 237–298 (Academic Press, 2008). https://doi.org/10.1016/B978-012374023-6.50012-9.

Hahn R: Comparison of protein A affinity sorbents, *J Chromatogr B* 790:35–51, 2003.

Jungbauer A: Continuous downstream processing of biopharmaceuticals, *Trends Biotechnol* 31:479–492, 2013.

Juza M, Mazzotti M, Morbidelli M: Simulated moving-bed chromatography and its application to chirotechnology, *Trends Biotechnol* 18:108–118, 2000.

Kasai K: Frontal affinity chromatography: a unique research tool for biospecific interaction that promotes glycobiology, *Proc Jpn Acad Ser B Phys Biol Sci* 90:215–234, 2014.

Kim TK, et al.: Experimental design of the multicolumn countercurrent solvent gradient purification (MCSGP) unit for the separation of PEGylated proteins, *Ind Eng Chem Res* 60:10764–10776, 2021.

Krättli M, Müller-Späth T, Morbidelli M: Multifraction separation in countercurrent chromatography (MCSGP), *Biotechnol Bioeng* 110:2436–2444, 2013.

Lin DQ, Zhang QL, Yao SJ: Model-assisted approaches for continuous chromatography: current situation and challenges, *J Chromatogr A* 1637, 2021.

Mahajan E, George A, Wolk B: Improving affinity chromatography resin efficiency using semi-continuous chromatography, *J Chromatogr A* 1227:154–162, 2012.

Makurvet FD: Biologics vs. small molecules: drug costs and patient access, *Med Drug Discov* 9, 2021, 100075.

Malik, M. I. & Pasch, H. Chapter 1—Basic principles of size exclusion and liquid interaction chromatography of polymers. in (eds. Malik, M. I., Mays, J. & Shah, M. R. B. T.-M. C. of Molecular characterization of polymers: a fundamental guide) 1–59 (Elsevier, 2021). doi: https://doi.org/10.1016/B978-0-12-819768-4.00007-5.

Mallik B, Chakravarti B, Chakravarti DN: Principles of chromatography, *Curr Protoc Essent Lab Tech* 2016:6.1.1–6.1.23, 2016.

Mathiasson L, et al.: *Scalable continuous chromatography process for enhanced efficiency in biomanufacturing*, 2020. Cytiva.

McCue JT: Chapter 25—Theory and use of hydrophobic interaction chromatography in protein purification applications, In Burgess RR, Deutscher MPBT-M, editors: *Guide to protein purification*, ed 2, vol. 463, 2009, Academic Press, pp 405–414.

Mukherjee S: Chapter 2—Isolation and purification of industrial enzymes: advances in enzyme technology, In Singh RS, Singhania RR, Pandey A, Larroche CBT-A, editors: *Biomass, biofuels, biochemicals*, 2019, Elsevier, pp 41–70. https://doi.org/10.1016/B978-0-444-64114-4.00002-9.

Müller-Späth T, StröHlein G, Lyngberg O, Maclean D: Enabling high purities and yields in therapeutic peptide purification using multicolumn countercurrent solvent gradient purification, *Chim Oggi/Chemistry Today* 31:56–60, 2013a.

Müller-Späth T, StröHlein G, Bavand M: Productivity boost for biopurification: twin-column ultra-high resolution chromatography, *Genet Eng Biotechnol News* 33, 2013b.

Müller-Späth T, et al.: Increasing capacity utilization in protein A chromatography, *BioPharm Int* 26:33–38, 2013c.

Najera M: Selecting a multicolumn chromatography solution, *Genet Eng Biotechnol News* 37:20–21, 2016.

Narayanan H, Sponchioni M, Morbidelli M: Integration and digitalization in the manufacturing of therapeutic proteins, *Chem Eng Sci* 248, 2022, 117159.

Nicoud R-M: The amazing ability of continuous chromatography to adapt to a moving environment, *Ind Eng Chem Res* 53:3755–3765, 2014.

Nuventra Pharma Sciences: *Points to consider in drug development of biologics and small molecules*, 2020, Nuventra Pharma Sciences, pp 1–11.

Ötes O, et al.: Scale-up of continuous multicolumn chromatography for the protein a capture step: from bench to clinical manufacturing, *J Biotechnol* 281:168–174, 2018.

Pfister D, Nicoud L, Morbidelli M: 2—Fundamentals of protein chromatography, In *Continuous biopharmaceutical processes: chromatography, conjugation, and protein stability*, 2018, Cambridge University Press, pp 27–83. https://doi.org/10.1017/9781108332897.003.

Poole, C. F. The essence of chromatography, Elsevier Science, 2003.

Rader RA: (Re)defining biopharmaceutical, *Nat Biotechnol* 26:743–751, 2008.

Reck JM, Pabst TM, Hunter AK, Carta G: Separation of antibody monomer-dimer mixtures by frontal analysis, *J Chromatogr A* 1500:96–104, 2017.

Rufer AC: Drug discovery for enzymes, *Drug Discov Today* 26:875–886, 2021.

Sartorius: *Protein A resin reduction achieved with process transfer from batch to BioSMB*, 2021. Bioprocess Online.

Shi C, Vogg S, Lin DQ, Sponchioni M, Morbidelli M: Analysis and optimal design of batch and two-column continuous chromatographic frontal processes for monoclonal antibody purification, *Biotechnol Bioeng* 15, 2021a. https://doi.org/10.1002/bit.27763.

Shi C, et al.: Process development and optimization of continuous capture with three-column periodic countercurrent chromatography, *Biotechnol Bioeng* 118:3313–3322, 2021b.

Shukla AA, Hubbard B, Tressel T, Guhan S, Low D: Downstream processing of monoclonal antibodies-Application of platform approaches, *J Chromatogr B Anal Technol Biomed Life Sci* 848:28–39, 2007.

Steinebach F, Müller-Späth T, Morbidelli M: Continuous countercurrent chromatography for capture and polishing steps in biopharmaceutical production, *Biotechnol J* 11:1126–1141, 2016.

Steinebach F, Ulmer N, Decker L, Aumann L, Morbidelli M: Experimental design of a twin-column countercurrent gradient purification process, *J Chromatogr A* 1492:19–26, 2017.

Ströhlein G, Aumann L, Mazzotti M, Morbidelli M: A continuous, countercurrent multi-column chromatographic process incorporating modifier gradients for ternary separations, *J Chromatogr A* 1126:338–346, 2006.

Ulmer N, Muller-spath T, Neunstoecklin B, Aumann L, Bavand M: Affinity capture of F(ab')2 fragments: using twin-column countercurrent chromatography, *Bioprocess Int* 13:22–29, 2015.

Ulmer N, Pfister D, Morbidelli M: Reactive separation processes for the production of PEGylated proteins, *Curr Opin Colloid Interface Sci* 31:86–91, 2017.

Utturkar A, et al.: A direct approach for process development using single column experiments results in predictable streamlined multi-column chromatography bioprocesses, *Biotechnol J* 14:1–23, 2019a.

Utturkar A, et al.: A direct approach for process development using single column experiments results in predictable streamlined multi-column chromatography bioprocesses, *Biotechnol J* 14, 2019b.

Veber DF, et al.: Molecular properties that influence the oral bioavailability of drug candidates, *J Med Chem* 45:2615–2623, 2002.

Vogg S, Ulmer N, Souquet J, Broly H, Morbidelli M: Experimental evaluation of the impact of intrinsic process parameters on the performance of a continuous chromatographic polishing unit (MCSGP), *Biotechnol J* 14:1–8, 2019.

Vogg S, Müller-Späth T, Morbidelli M: Design space and robustness analysis of batch and countercurrent frontal chromatography processes for the removal of antibody aggregates, *J Chromatogr A* 1619:12–14, 2020.

Walsh G: Biopharmaceutical benchmarks 2018, *Nat Biotechnol* 36:1136–1145, 2018.

Wang Y, Teraoka I, Hansen FY, Peters GH, Hassager O: A theoretical study of the separation principle in size exclusion chromatography, *Macromolecules* 43:1651–1659, 2010.

Yang YJ, Lee CH, Koo YM: Separation of amino acids by simulated moving bed using competitive langmuir isotherm, *Biotechnol Bioprocess Eng* 9:331, 2004.

CHAPTER THREE

# Application of Multicolumn Countercurrent Solvent Gradient Purification to the polishing of therapeutic proteins

**Martina Catani* and Chiara De Luca**
Department of Chemical, Pharmaceutical and Agricultural Sciences, University of Ferrara, Ferrara, Italy
*Corresponding author: e-mail address: ctnmtn@unife.it

## Contents



## Abstract

Industrial purification of biopharmaceuticals is usually performed through single-column preparative liquid chromatography. The polishing step, which is required to remove all product-related impurities, represents one of the most critical points of the entire production process of biopharmaceuticals. Indeed, product-related impurities have very similar chemical characteristics to the target compound. The removal of these impurities via chromatography is very challenging, because also their chromatographic behavior is like that of the target. It follows that, despite the use of very shallow gradients to increase resolution of critical impurities, chromatograms are very often characterized by overlapping regions where target and impurities coelute (center-cut separations). This results in an intrinsic limitation of single-column processes that is the so-called yield-purity trade-off.

*Advances in Chemical Engineering*, Volume 59
ISSN 0065-2377
https://doi.org/10.1016/bs.ache.2022.03.003

This drawback can be partially overcome thanks to the use of multicolumn continuous (or semicontinuous) techniques. In particular, this chapter is focused on the advantages of Multicolumn Countercurrent Solvent Gradient Purification (MCSGP), one of the most recently developed countercurrent approaches specifically designed for challenging center-cut separations. The automatic internal recycling of the impure fractions inside the chromatographic system results in an increased yield without compromising the purity of the pool besides allowing for the automatization of the process. Each step of the purification process will be illustrated, together with a synthetic overview of most interesting applications of MCSGP.

## 1. Introduction

In the last decade, protein-based therapeutics have increasingly become an important class of drugs in the pharmaceutical industry. Their success is attributable to their unique properties, including high specificity and high potency as well as reduced toxic side effects (Yin et al., 2015). These characteristics make them clearly advantageous over common synthetic small molecules drugs, which are generally associated with significant side effects and generation of harmful metabolites. In addition, improvements in recombinant DNA technology have allowed to obtain therapeutic proteins with different properties to treat a wide variety of diseases, including cancers, autoimmunity, inflammations, exposure to infectious agents, and genetic disorders.

The number of approved protein-based drugs has tremendously increased since the introduction of the first one (human insulin derived from recombinant DNA) in 1982. Currently, it is estimated that almost 40–50% of the products under development are biopharmaceuticals, most of which are based on therapeutic proteins (Walsh, 2018).

Protein based drugs can be classified in three distinct ways. The first one is based on their molecular type, so one can distinguish between blood factors, antibody-based drugs, enzymes, engineered protein scaffolds, Fc fusion proteins, hormones, interferons, interleukins, anticoagulants, bone morphogenetic proteins and thrombolytics (Carter, 2011).

Another classification is based on their pharmacological activity which allows to group therapeutic proteins into five classes: (i) replacing proteins which are abnormal of deficient; (ii) augmenting an existing pathway; (iii) providing novel functions or activities; (iv) interfering with other molecules or organisms; (v) delivering other compounds or proteins (i.e., radionuclides, cytotoxic drugs, effector proteins) (Leader et al., 2008).

Finally, therapeutic proteins can be divided into three groups according to the molecular mechanism: (i) specific noncovalent binders, including monoclonal antibodies (mAbs), Fc fusion proteins and polyclonal immunoglobulins as well as other numerous proteins such as Human follicle-stimulating hormone (FSH), Growth hormone (GH), Salmon calcitonin, etc.; (ii) protein interacting with covalent bonds, such as lactase, trypsin, papain, antithrombin III, etc. and (iii) others (e.g., human serum albumin, which is used to increase plasma osmolarity) (Dimitrov, 2012).

## 2. Production of therapeutic proteins

Production of protein-based therapeutics (and in general of biopharmaceuticals) can be divided into two parts: the *upstream processing*, where the protein is produced by living organisms and the *downstream processing*, where a series of purification steps are performed in order to meet purity specifications for pharmaceutical scopes as illustrated in Fig. 1.

### 2.1 Upstream processing

Therapeutic proteins are commonly produced by means of recombinant approaches involving different systems including bacteria, yeasts, fungi, as well as transgenic plants and animals. However, the number of host cells industrially used is quite limited. Among the most widely employed systems,

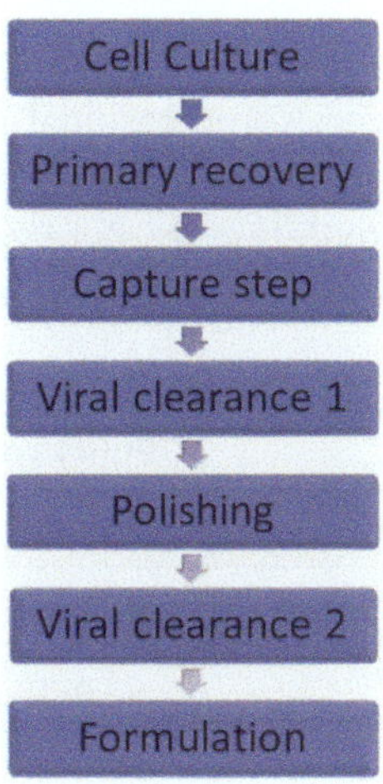


**Fig. 1** Scheme reporting the typical steps of a bioprocess to produce therapeutic proteins.

it is worth mentioning: (i) *E. coli* bacterial strain, which is a versatile and nonexpensive system; (ii) *Saccharomyces cerevisiae* and *Pichia pastoris* yeast cells which have been successfully applied for the expression of insulin and albumin; (iii) mammalian cell cultures from *Chinese Hamster Ovary* (CHO), which are currently the most popular ones to produce most protein-based therapeutics (and, especially, monoclonal antibodies). Indeed, despite their complexity, this kind of cells are preferred over other hosts (e.g., bacteria, plants yeast) since they allow a better protein folding, assembly, and posttranslational modifications (e.g., glycosylation).

## 2.2 Process- and product-related impurities

Even though often highly selective, all production methods lead to complex mixtures where the target protein is present together with a series of other species (impurities). These "unwanted" chemicals need to be removed during the downstream processing in order to isolate the target protein with an acceptable purity level for pharmaceutical scopes. In particular, the impurities can be classified into two groups (de Luca et al., 2020b; de Luca et al., 2021b; Pfister et al., 2018):

- Process-related impurities originating from the production process itself such as nutrient media, salts, pieces of host cells or of DNA, viruses, etc. or chemical modifications to the product (e.g., PEGylation)
- Product-related impurities which are species chemically similar to the target product (e.g., isoforms, fragments, protein variants, aggregates, etc.)

These species are usually almost entirely removed during the downstream purification process; however, some residual amount may be left within the bulk drug substance. Table 1 reports some approximated purity specifications, even if it is difficult to define absolute values applicable to all kind of biopharmaceuticals since they depend on the type of drug, dose, and usage.

**Table 1** Typical purity specifications for protein-based drugs.

| Species | Purity specification |
|---|---|
| Target protein content | >99.9% |
| Aggregates | <1 ppm |
| Ligand leakage | <1 ppm |
| Virus content | Absence (probability $<10^{-9}$) |
| DNA content | <10 pg/dose |

Among the impurities reported in Table 1, aggregates need to be accurately monitored since they can induce immune reactions or other dangerous side effects. The presence of viruses needs to be also carefully evaluated but since their complete removal is not possible, some limits are suggested by the World Health Organization (WHO). For instance, in the case of vaccines one adverse case in $10^9$ doses is accepted (which corresponds to a probability of $10^{-9}$). Other types of critical impurities include leakage of ligands or other chemicals from chromatographic media and DNA content.

Finally, as previously mentioned, most therapeutic proteins are not produced as a single molecular entity but rather as a series of variants and isoforms which, despite their similar molecular structure, can drastically have different biological and pharmacological activity; therefore, it is important to maintain their distribution within acceptable limits.

## 2.3 Downstream processing

The first step of the downstream processing is a *primary recovery* (see Fig. 1) of the target protein from the cell culture broth. It usually consists in the separation of the supernatant from the cells and cells debris which form during cell autolysis by means of centrifugation or filtration (Liu et al., 2010). If the protein is expressed extracellularly then it will be isolated by collecting the broth supernatant. This is usually done when mammalian cells are used (the process takes the name of *clarification*). On the other hand, if expression occurs in the extracellular volume, the protein of interest is collected after having removed the supernatant and after cell disruption. In any case, primary recovery is a relatively simple step due to the different size of proteins and cells.

The fluid collected is then further processed since it contains many impurities. In downstream processes, preparative liquid chromatography is by far the most employed technique due to its numerous advantages: it is flexible, versatile and selective, and can distinguish between molecules showing different size, charge or hydrophobicity. Moreover, if proper working conditions are chosen, it is possible to modulate, to some extent, the separation between similar species. Generally, however, it is quite complex to separate at the baseline large biomolecules, even when more than one different chromatographic modes are used consecutively, as it will be illustrated in the next sections (de Luca et al., 2020b; Tarafder et al., 2010).

Just after the primary recovery, a *capture step* is usually applied whose scope is to extract the maximum amount of the target protein from the feed and to remove process-related impurities as much as possible. Since these species are chemically different to the target protein, approaches based on affinity chromatography are commonly applied. These methods rely on the use of adsorbents functionalized with natural or synthetic ligands that allow to establish highly specific reversible interaction with the protein of interest. For instance, stationary phases functionalized with Protein A are commonly used for the purification of antibodies, since specific interactions are established between the Fc portions of immunoglobulin G (IgG) and Protein A (Curling, 2008; Hober et al., 2007). Among the other ligands, it is worth mentioning heparin to isolate plasma proteins (Burnouf and Radosevich, 2001) and recombinant factor VII (Knäblein, 2013).

After the capture step, one or more *polishing steps* are required in order to remove process-related impurities. Since these species are molecular variants of the target proteins (e.g., aggregates, deamidates, truncates, isoforms, etc.) their removal is particularly challenging since also their chromatographic behavior will be like that of the target. Therefore, ion exchange chromatography (IEX) or ion-pair reversed-phase liquid chromatography (IP-RPLC) are generally employed associated with the use of very shallow gradients. In addition, size-exclusion chromatography can be also effective for removing aggregates.

Another important step of the downstream processing is *viral clearance* to remove residuals form viruses. Different approaches can be adopted to this end, including low-pH inactivation, heat inactivation, filtration, solvents/detergents treatment and gamma irradiation (Remington, 2015).

Then, a *formulation step* occurs to achieve the target protein at the appropriate composition and concentration allowing for a proper drug delivery into the organism. Usually, the drug is dissolved in buffered solutions (at a fixed pH) containing also other excipients such as salts, surfactants, etc. Typically, diafiltration (DF) or ultrafiltration (UF) are performed to exchange the buffer and to increase concentration of the target protein, respectively. The biomanufacturing process usually ends with a sterile *filtration step* and other *fill/finish operations* (Curling, 2008; Houp, 2009).

## 3. Relevant parameters for the evaluation of purification processes

Batch and continuous processes are usually evaluated in terms of relevant parameters that are determined by analyzing the eluted fractions by means of a proper high performance liquid chromatography (HPLC) analytical method.

The most important parameter is purity of the target compound which is essential for pharmaceutical scopes. It is calculated as the ratio between the area of the target product and the total area of all the peaks detected by analytical HPLC. In MCSGP it is calculated as the mean of the purities of all the pools referred to the steady-state (see Section 5.3):

$$\text{Purity}\,\% = \frac{A_{\text{product}}}{A_{\text{total}}} \times 100$$

Another relevant parameter, particularly important in the case of very expensive biopharma, is yield (or recovery) of the entire purification process. It is defined as the ratio of the mass of the target product in collected pool and the mass of the product from the feed injected into the column:

$$\text{Recovery}\,\% = \frac{m_{\text{prod collected}}}{m_{\text{prod injected}}} \times 100$$

The third parameter in order of importance is productivity of the process which indicates how much target molecule is produces per minute and per column volume ($V_{col}$). It is expressed as the mass of the target product collected in the purified pool per total volume of stationary phase and per time:

$$\text{Productivity}\left(\frac{\text{g}}{\text{L h}}\right) = \frac{m_{\text{prod collected}}}{n \times V_{\text{col}} \times \text{time}}$$

where $n$ is the number of columns used ($n = 1$ for single-column processes; $n \geq 2$ in MCSGP), whereas the time considered is the duration of a run in batch conditions or a cycle in MCSGP.

Finally, another aspect that is considered is solvent consumption that is defined as the volume of eluent required to collect the desired quantity of purified product:

$$\text{Solvent consumption (L/g)} = \frac{V_{\text{solvent}}}{m_{\text{prod collected}}}$$

## 4. Limitations of batch chromatography

As already said, the aim of the polishing steps is to remove to a great extent the product-related impurities, having a structure very similar to the target product, in order to obtain a product with acceptable purity.

Examples of product-related impurities in proteins samples are aggregates, incorrectly modified or unfolded proteins, whereas regarding peptides they can be truncated or deamidated species or amino acid chains where an amino acid inserts in the wrong position or does not react completely. The polishing processing is the last phase in the manufacturing of Active Pharmaceuticals Ingredients (APIs), before the drug is prepared in its final formulation (as emulsion, encapsulated, for oral use, etc.) and marketed.

Traditionally, polishing processes are performed in batch conditions, i.e., with the use of a single column. In batch liquid chromatography, the sample injected is completely eluted before the next injection is performed, and between two consecutive injections the column is cleaned and regenerated.

Very frequently gradient elution chromatography is used, where all the components adsorb onto the stationary phase before gradually eluting by means of a solvent gradient. The order of elution is correlated to the different affinity of every species for the stationary and mobile phases, since the retention of biomolecules is profoundly affected by the mobile phase composition (e.g., content of salt, fraction of organic modifier). Beside the nonspecificity of adsorption, another aspect must be considered, namely the fact that on pilot or industrial scale the purification is performed under preparative, nonlinear conditions. The amount of sample injected is chosen to overload the column until a compromise between purity, yield and productivity is reached. High volumes of feed to be purified are injected for every run, and this, together with the nonspecific adsorption, results in peaks not well resolved. The overlap situation worsens with increasing the mass loaded. The outcome of the separation, namely the resolution of the main peak from close-eluting species, has an impact on the performance of the purification process and, as a consequence, improving the resolution is mandatory to enhance the process performance, even though it is a challenging task.

The target peak elutes as intermediate between two other groups of impurities, that are respectively more weakly and more strongly adsorbed, with which it overlaps on the front and on the tail (Aumann and Morbidelli, 2007; Chibério et al., 2020; Müller-Späth et al., 2013).

Only a narrow region of the main peak is pure enough to fulfill the purity requirements, but this results in a low recovery, since an important amount of target lies in the overlapping regions. Consequently, collecting a considerable amount of pure product is nearly impossible. The other option is to broaden the collection region, which results in an improved yield at the expense of the purity, since also some impurities are pooled with the product. Therefore, when using batch chromatography, this dual behavior

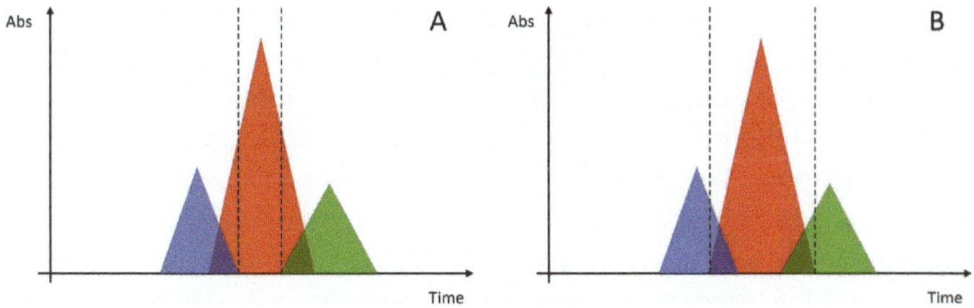


**Fig. 2** Schematic representation of the yield-purity trade-off. The red peak is the target product, eluting between two groups of close-eluting impurities, more weakly adsorbed (blue peak) and more strongly adsorbed (green peak). Narrow collection window leads to higher purity but lower recovery, since a part of the product is discarded (A); broad collection window leads to high recovery but low purity, since also a portion of impurities peaks is collected (B). *Reproduced with permission from de Luca C, Lievore G, Bozza D, et al: Downstream processing of therapeutic peptides by means of preparative liquid chromatography,* Molecules *26:1–20, 2021. doi:10.3390/molecules26154688.*

translates into a yield-purity trade-off, a limit intrinsic to batch processes according to which it is not possible to achieve a high purity and a high yield at the same time (see Fig. 2).

The overlapping regions can be discarded, with a consistent and unjustified waste of expensive product, or recycled, meaning reprocessed and purified again, manually by the operator, or automatically, through a commuting recycling valve. This makes single-column chromatography sometimes impractical and not very productive.

To solve this drawback, some options can be considered. A possible one would be to decrease the mass loaded into the column on the one side, or the gradient slope on the other side. This choice, nevertheless, would lead to longer times (and therefore lower productivity) and higher solvent consumption. Otherwise, more efficient columns can be employed, with smaller particles size, leading however to excessively high backpressures. In conclusion, these options are not feasible solutions to the problem (Steinebach et al., 2017b; Vogg et al., 2019).

An attractive alternative is to replace single-column processes with countercurrent chromatography. The term countercurrent refers to a class of chromatographic processes in which the stationary and the mobile phase move in two opposite directions. Except for True Moving Bed, the movement of the stationary phase is not real but simulated through the switching of the inlet and outlet valves of the columns (Müller-Späth et al., 2010; Pfister et al., 2018).

The countercurrent movement of two phases is widely adopted in biological systems, such as in mammals and other animals, to exchange heat in the blood, to change the concentration of a component in a biological fluid, etc., and this mechanism has been taken as a model by countercurrent chromatography. The potentiality of countercurrent reveals when compounds contained in the same feed, with different affinity for the mobile and stationary phases, are to be separated. The compounds with similar affinity to the mobile phase, which would be earlier eluting, barely adsorb on the stationary phase and follow the path of the eluent. On the other hand, compounds which interact more strongly with the stationary phase (more retained ones) adsorb on it and thus move in the opposite directions, from which the term *countercurrent*. Usually, the target compound elutes between two other groups of impurities, one more and one less retained respectively, therefore, by exploiting the countercurrent principle, a better separation between them can be reached. As a consequence, a window of the main peak results to be pure and can be immediately collected, whereas the front and the tail do not fulfill purity requirements yet and must be recycled within the same unit.

What is important is to understand is whether and in which cases continuous multicolumn processes can perform better than single-column chromatography. They are particularly appealing for separations requiring a large number of theoretical plates (meaning characterized by low selectivity but aiming at high purity and recovery) and exhibiting remarkable mass transfer limitations. In recycling chromatography, the target compound contained in the overlapping regions is reintroduced into the following column just after being eluted from the first one. Each passage through the columns increases the number of theoretical plates that the compounds experience and enhances chromatographic resolution. The greatest improvements are related to the possibility to reduce the number of plates necessary to achieve a target separation performance, which is associated with a decrease in column length and an increase in mobile phase velocity. In protein polishing, this leads to an improvement in the performance, such as an increase in the recovery at a high purity, and to a greater resin utilization, even though this comes at the expense of the hardware complexity (Baur et al., 2016). When engineering developments lead to a technology which is more efficient and which allows to cut the overall costs by reshaping already existing operation schemes, an *intensification* of the process is obtained (Gerstweiler et al., 2021; Segovia-Hernández and Bonilla-Petriciolet, 2016). Process intensification through continuous manufacturing allows to avoid hold steps, which do not represent value added and are detrimental for unstable or labile components. For example, some peptides and proteins tend to aggregate, to form fibrils or gel quite rapidly (Zapadka et al., 2017).

Moreover, it simplifies the process with positive returns also in terms of productivity and solvent consumption and, as a consequence, on the whole process footprint (Gjoka et al., 2017; Warikoo et al., 2012).

To perform countercurrent chromatography, multicolumn units are needed, meaning instruments equipped with two or more columns, identical in terms of column and particle geometry and functionalization, so that the feed can be continuously or semicontinuously injected into the system either in one column or in another (Gerstweiler et al., 2021). If the unit is equipped with two or three columns, the system works semicontinuously because during some steps the feed is not being introduced into the columns, whereas if the columns are six the process is continuous, since at every moment the sample is fed in one of the columns. Multicolumn continuous chromatographic approaches have become more and more appealing in the field of purification of high value biopharmaceuticals, especially proteins and peptides, since they allow to overcome the trade-off typical of batch methods, with economic repercussions as well. The amplitude of the economic gains is, however, product- and process-specific (Girard et al., 2015). The equipment is also compact, which is fundamental to flexible manufacturing and to the accommodation of dynamic market demand.

Initially, in the 1950s, the only continuous chromatographic process developed was Simulated Moving Bed (SMB), which however could only separate binary mixtures under isocratic conditions (Mazzotti et al., 1997; Schramm et al., 2003). Different versions of this technique have been proposed during the years, but its applications are still limited to isocratic separations of two components, which is not the case of proteins polishing. Indeed, proteins and peptides mixtures contain a large number of variants and impurities whose retention can be modulated by varying the mobile phase composition along the chromatographic run by means of a gradient. The use of a gradient, anyway, is not compatible with SMB.

Multicolumn Countercurrent Solvent Gradient Purification (MCSGP) is a continuous process carried out in linear gradient conditions and designed for challenging ternary separations where many product-related impurities are present. Its strength points are the automation of the process and the internal recycling of the impure fractions eluting, which are reprocessed inside the unit thanks to a system of valves. Also, it has been developed to work in gradient conditions (Müller-Späth and Morbidelli, 2015), which is of utmost importance when dealing with biomolecules (de Luca et al., 2020a; Grossmann et al., 2010; Krättli et al., 2013), and, as already said, it cannot be done with other continuous techniques.

In the following, MCSGP operating principles and its applications will be reviewed.

# 5. Theory of Multicolumn Countercurrent Solvent Gradient Purification

## 5.1 Starting point: The batch run

Before explaining the operating principles of MCSGP, a deep description of the batch process must be provided. The case of interest is the so-called center-cut or ternary separation, where, as already stated above, the target peak coelutes on the front and on the rear side with close-eluting impurities. Batch processes can be decomposed in three phases: sample loading, gradient elution and regeneration of the stationary phase. However, four tasks can be recognized within the gradient elution, for a total of six tasks, as it can be seen in Fig. 3.

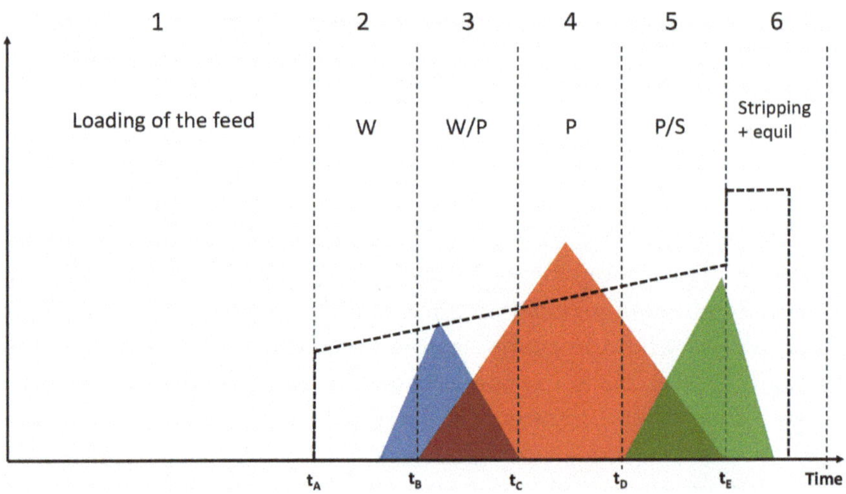


**Fig. 3** Schematic representation of the tasks accomplished during a batch run in gradient conditions. The widths of the windows 2–5 are generally different. *Reproduced with permission from de Luca C, Felletti S, Lievore G, et al: Modern trends in downstream processing of biotherapeutics through continuous chromatography: the potential of multicolumn countercurrent solvent gradient purification,* Trends Analyt Chem *132, 2020b. doi:10.1016/j.trac.2020.116051.*

Particularly, the different regions of the chromatogram are the following:

1. the equilibrated column is loaded with fresh feed. The components adsorb on the stationary phase and, after that, the gradient can start;
2. at the beginning of the gradient, only the group of weakly adsorbed impurities (W), which are the least retained on the resin, elutes;
3. at some point, together with W, also some product (P) starts eluting. This is the first overlapping zone, where the product does not satisfy the purity requirement because of the presence of W, but at the same time it cannot be wasted, otherwise the yield would dramatically worsen;
4. In the following region, product eluting is highly pure and can be collected without further purification procedures;
5. this is the second overlapping zone, where P partially overlap with strongly adsorbed impurities (S), that begin to elute at this point;
6. at the end of the gradient, very retained impurities are to be completely washed out through the stripping of the column, which is also reequilibrated.

Therefore, zone 4 represents the collection region whereas windows 3 and 5 are the ones to be recycled. To obtain the concentration profile of the product and, when possible, also of W and S impurities, fractions are collected along the gradient and analyzed through an HPLC method. With this offline analysis, also the purity profile can be plotted as a function of time. The yield is calculated based on the product amount contained in each fraction, with respect to the mass injected.

In Fig. 3, the six zones are defined by some specific times, named characteristic times, which are needed to set the MCSGP process, as it will be explained later.

## 5.2 Working principles of MCSGP

When transferring a method from batch to continuous, the same steps just described for the batch must be accomplished. The difference is that, in order to transform this sequence of steps into a continuous procedure, the tasks that would be performed in the single-column at different times, now are accomplished into different columns simultaneously.

In principle, as many columns as the zones identified in the chromatogram could be used, with each column attaining a different task. In its former version, the unit consisted of six columns, but then it has been more and more simplified toward a reduction in the number of columns. Nowadays, MCSGP can be run even using only two columns, with a consequent simplification in the connections and in the microfluidics (Aumann and Morbidelli, 2006; Aumann et al., 2007; Müller-Späth et al., 2013; Steinebach et al., 2017b).

If the number of columns is smaller than the number of zones in Fig. 3, every column must perform successively different tasks that previously were accomplished at the same time into different columns. This means that, at some times, some tasks are not performed into the instrument: for example, the feed cannot be loaded continuously, and this step becomes intermittent.

The MCSGP alternates between steps involving the columns working in parallel, during the pooling and the regeneration steps, and steps where the columns work in series, to adsorb and recycle the impure product. Therefore, in the first case the columns work disconnected as in batch, in an open-loop configuration, since the eluent must leave the system, whereas, in the second case, the columns are interconnected in order for the eluent to be redirected into the following column and recycled.

The loading step in MCSGP differs from the batch, as it can be seen by comparing Figs. 3 and 4. Indeed, while in batch the sample is loaded in a

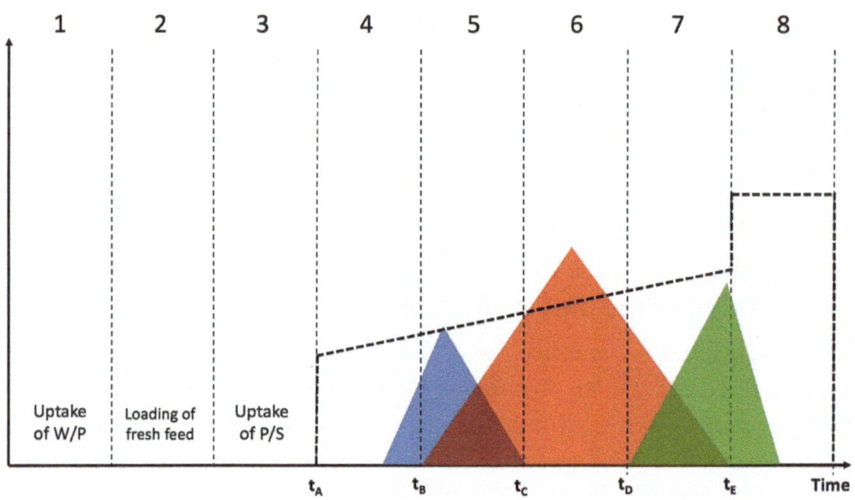


**Fig. 4** Schematic diagram of the zones that can be identified in twin-column MCSGP. The tasks accomplished in each zone is also described representing the connection between the two columns. *Modified with permission from de Luca C, Felletti S, Lievore G, et al: From batch to continuous chromatographic purification of a therapeutic peptide through multicolumn countercurrent solvent gradient purification.* J Chromatogr A *1625, 2020a. doi:10.1016/j.chroma.2020.461304.*

single phase, in MCSGP it is loaded in three phases in the column of interest: a certain amount of product derives from the recycling of the overlapping region W/P coming from another column (zone 1 in Fig. 4), then some fresh feed is added (zone 2 in Fig. 4), and finally the overlapping region P/S eluting from another column is loaded (zone 3 in Fig. 4). The total amount of target compound loaded per gram of stationary phase is kept constant in the two processes. Besides the three loading steps, the other five steps are the same as the batch, with the exception that the overlapping regions (which now are zones 5 and 7 in Fig. 4) do not leave the unit but are redirected toward another column.

In Fig. 5 the countercurrent principle subtended to the MCSGP technology is graphically illustrated. To run the process continuously, at some point each column switches one position to the left, and so on and so forth until they have completed all eight tasks. On the other side, the windows to be recycled move in the other direction, toward right (e.g., from position 5 to 1 or from 7 to 3). After a column has completed the series of eight tasks, from position 8 it goes back to position 1, and a cycle is completed. Along the positions occupied by each column after the loading and during the gradient, the concentration of organic modifier, meaning of the mobile phase component which drives elution, increases with the position number. However, when the overlapping regions are countercurrent recycled, they are loaded into a column containing a lower concentration of modifier, and therefore they require to be inline diluted with a

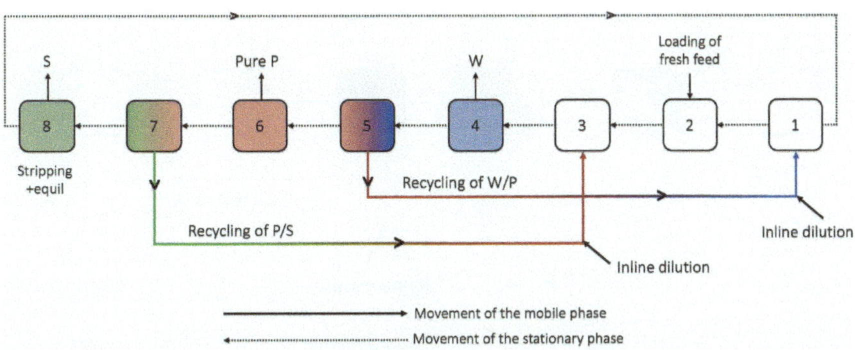


**Fig. 5** The countercurrent movement of the stationary and mobile phases is represented with colored (mobile phase) and dotted (stationary phase) arrows. Each column switches position moving to the left, while the overlapping windows are recycled into another column to the right. The positions enumerated in this scheme represent the steps described in the batch chromatogram, in Fig. 4.

compensation buffer, in order for the components to readsorb. So, a stream of mobile phase with low content of organic modifier is mixed with the overlapping regions during every recycling step, as shown in Fig. 5.

Theoretically, this sequence would require eight columns, one for each position. Nevertheless, the process can be carried out also on six, three or even two columns. Let us consider the case with six columns. The countercurrent principle is the same, but in some positions two tasks are fulfilled at the same time: in position 2, some fresh feed is injected, and W impurities elute and are discarded; in position 3, the recycling window W/P leaves the system while P/S enters into the column. Even in this case, the stationary phase moves toward left while the mobile phase toward right (see Fig. 6).

The configuration with six positions depicted in Fig. 6 can be performed even with three columns. In that case, the three columns work in an interconnected way when they occupy positions 1-3-5, since the eluent coming from position 5 enters the column in position 3 and the eluent eluting from position 3 goes into column 1; they work disconnected in positions 2-4-6, where they are loaded with feed, are collecting the purified product, and are regenerated respectively. Three-column MCSGP is a semicontinuous process since the feed is loaded into the instrument not continuously but intermittently (Fig. 7).

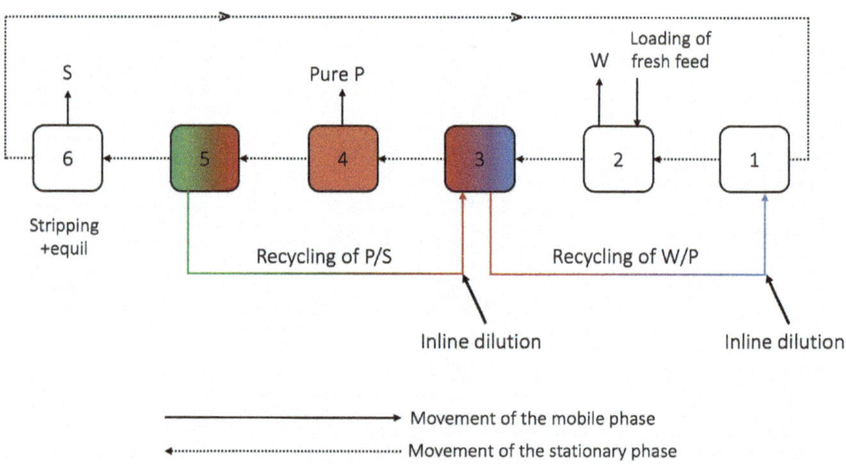


**Fig. 6** Countercurrent movement of stationary and mobile phases in the six-column MCSGP. The tasks are the same as in Fig. 5, but positions 2 and 3 account for two tasks each.

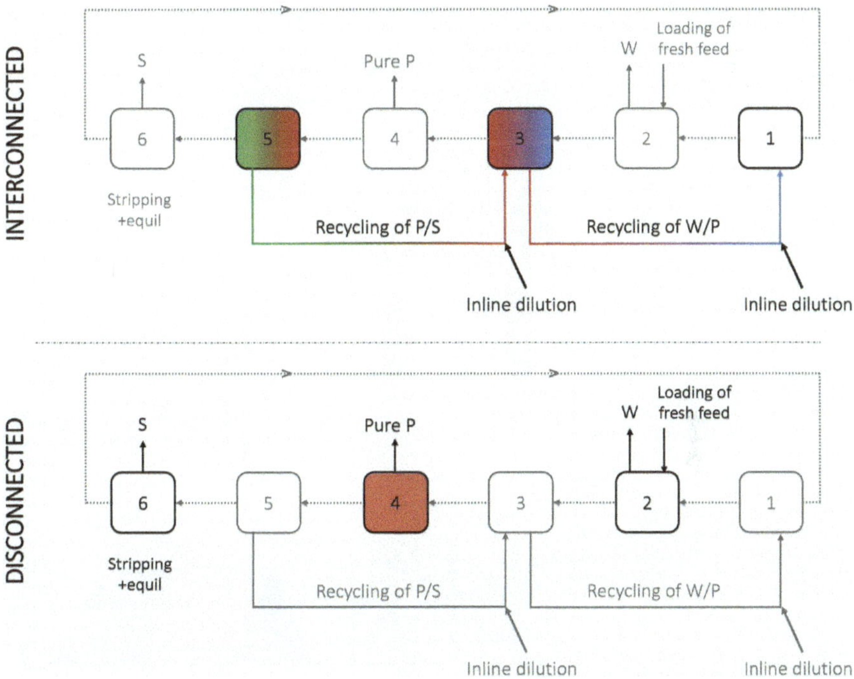


**Fig. 7** Relative positions of the columns in three-columns MCSGP. The possible configurations are the columns being interconnected (during the recycling) or disconnected (during the loading, collection, and regeneration).

The simplest configuration of the MCSGP process, as already stated above, is the twin-column version, where only two identical columns are used. To explain how they operate, the scheme in Fig. 8 must be considered, which harks back to the schemes in Figs. 4 and 5.

Let us consider Fig. 8, which represents two-column MCSGP process at the moment when column-1 receives the overlapping regions from column-2. The receiving column is said to be in *downstream* position, whereas the column from which the recycling windows elute is said to be in *upstream* position. Pointing the attention to column-1, it can be seen that when it is in position 1 it is receiving the W/P region coming from column-2, which is in position 5. In this step they are interconnected. Then they disconnect: column-1 is loaded with fresh feed, while from column-2 pure product elutes and can be collected. Then they connect again for the uptake of P/S zone into column-1 (position 3), while column-2 is accomplishing task n°7. After that, column-2 can be stripped, cleaned and regenerated, to get ready to receive again the sample to be purified. On the contrary, in column-1 (task 4) the

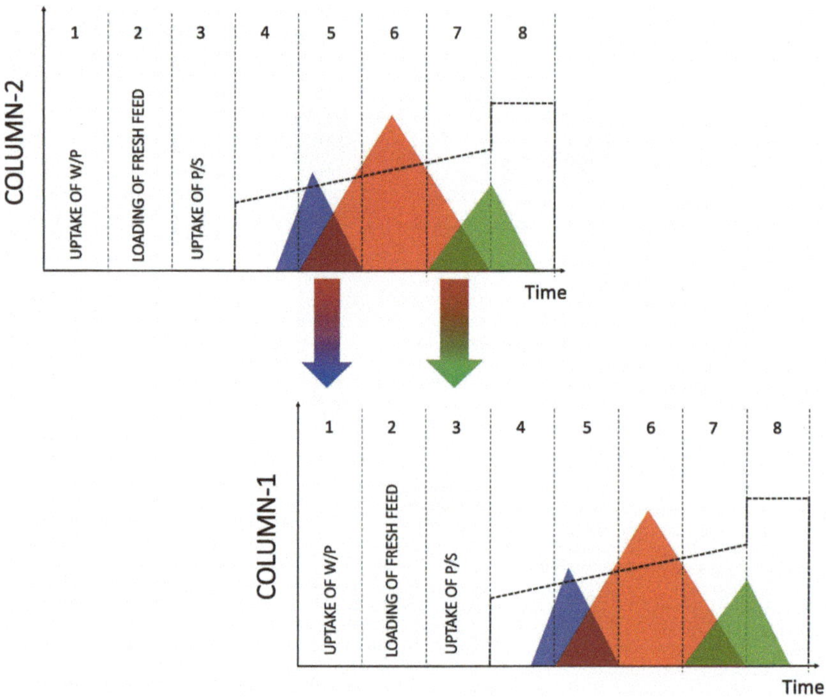


**Fig. 8** Scheme of the two-column MCSGP process. The tasks of the two columns are shifted of four positions at every time. The numeration of the columns is arbitrary.

solvent gradient can start, and W impurities are discarded. In the following, when W/P start eluting from column-1, it is redirected to column-2. At this point, column-1 is in position 5 and column-2 in position-1: they have exchanged position with respect to the beginning of the process. At every moment of the run, the columns are achieving tasks shifted of four positions, corresponding to half a cycle. Half a cycle is called a *switch*. Fig. 9 shows more in detail the connections between the columns and the tasks carried out by each column during one switch of the process. When the columns exchange again positions, meaning after two switches, a cycle is completed. Given the flow rate during the gradient, the durations of the different tasks are not the same. Nevertheless, in MCSGP the columns must always work in a coordinated and synchronized manner so that their valves can switch position at the same moment, therefore the flow rates of the different steps are not identical. What is important is that the volumes of mobile phase eluted within every step is kept equal between batch and MCSGP, and that's why, often, the X axes of the chromatogram (e.g., Figs. 3 and 4), instead of time, reports the elution volume, expressed as Column Volumes (CVs).

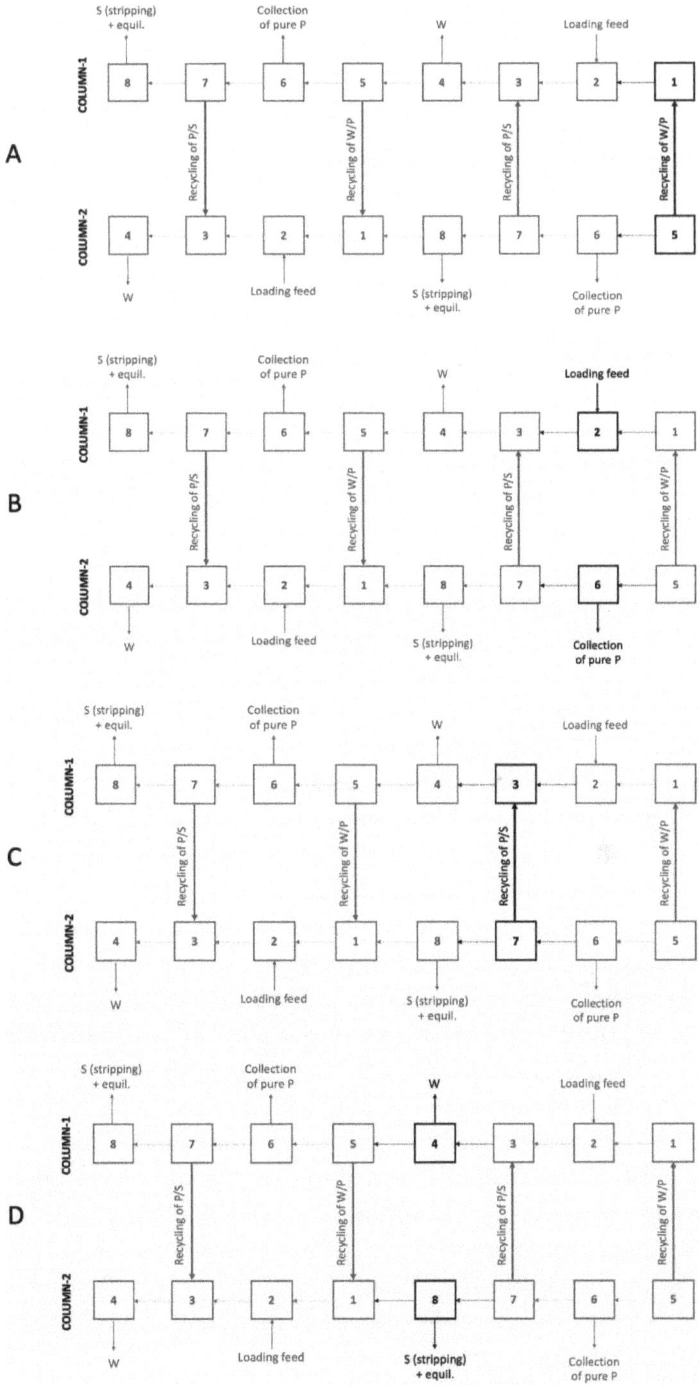


**Fig. 9** Example of a switch where column-1 is in downstream position (it is being loaded) where column-2 is in upstream position (it is experiencing the gradient elution). The four tasks fulfilled by each column and constituting the switch are shown (in order from A to D).

Even in the case of two-column MCSGP, there are moments where the feed is not being loaded, and therefore this process is semicontinuous.

## 5.3 Set-up of the MCSGP process

The first step to plan an MCSGP process is the development of a suitable batch method. This batch is named *design batch chromatogram* because it will be transferred to the continuous technology. It is generally selected based on the presence of a window in the chromatogram where the purity specifications are fulfilled, even if with a low yield.

Let us consider Fig. 3, for instance, which corresponds to a scheme of a hypothetical batch chromatogram, where the red peak (product) is not completely resolved from the blue one and the green one, representing not two single impurities but two groups of impurities. The steps occurring during the batch run have already been described. Focusing on the gradient, the recycling, wasting, and collection windows are chosen based on the fractions collected along the gradient and analyzed offline. The first step when it comes to the design procedure is to define the five regions during the elution (W, W/P, P, P/S, S), meaning to define their boundaries. In Fig. 3, these boundaries are indicated with five times from $t_A$ to $t_E$, called *characteristic times*. They are defined arbitrarily after the calculation of the so-called *Pareto curve*. This diagram reports purity as a function of yield and it is a graphical representation of the yield-purity trade-off which has already been mentioned above. To obtain this chart, the offline HPLC analysis of the fractions eluting during the gradient, with a different value of purity and recovery each, are needed. The first fraction to consider is the purest one, which is expected to show a low recovery. It must be imagined pooling it together with the purest one between its two neighboring fractions. The pool obtained shows a higher recovery but a lower purity than the purest fraction. Then, the same procedure is applied with this new pool: it is virtually pooled with the purest fraction among its two adjacent ones; again, the purity is decreasing, and the recovery is increasing. This operation is repeated until all the fractions containing the product have been pooled together and, theoretically, corresponds to broadening the collection window. The values of recovery and purity found for every pooling window are then plotted to determine the Pareto curve.

When $N$ fractions are pooled together, the total recovery of the pool is simply the sum of the recovery of every fraction:

$$\text{Recovery}_N\ (\%) = \sum_{i}^{N} \text{Recovery}_i$$

whereas the total purity is the sum of the purity of every fraction weighed for its recovery:

$$\text{Purity}_N\ (\%) = \frac{\sum_i^N \text{Recovery}_i \times \text{Purity}_i}{\sum_i^N \text{Recovery}_i}$$

This is because the contribution to the purity given by every fraction depends also on the product amount contained in it.

The upper point of the Pareto curve, located on the left, corresponds to the fraction with higher purity, while the lowest point on the right represents the purity that would be obtained if the whole product peak was collected (with a recovery around 100%). The trade-off lies in the worsening of one performance when improving the other.

A qualitative example of a Pareto curve is shown in Fig. 10.

Once the Pareto curve is plotted, a point on it must be chosen which satisfies the purity requirements and shows a quite high recovery. This point corresponds to a pool of fractions that is taken as a first trial for the collection window when transferring the method to MCSGP. The times defining the beginning and the end of this fractions pool are taken as $t_C$ and $t_D$. The time where the gradient starts is taken as $t_A$. $t_B$ and $t_E$ are chosen more arbitrarily and they are selected in order to minimize the amount of product wasted in the waste windows (zone 2 and 6 of Fig. 3). Fig. 3 corresponds to the ideal case where no product is discarded in regions 2 and 6. Unfortunately, this is hard to obtain: in order to avoid an accumulation, cycle by cycle, of the impurities in the pooling window due to overloading effects causing fronting or tailing, working conditions are selected to "play safe." Therefore, it is preferable to waste some product in the wasting regions than to contaminate the product pool with accumulating impurities.

The times $t_A$–$t_E$ (Figs. 3 and 4) are used to set the cyclic MCSGP process, and specifically represent the times where the inlet and outlet column valves switch position to connect or disconnect the columns. If no accumulation occurs, after a few cycles the UV profile stabilizes and does not change anymore cycle by cycle. Also, for every pool collected (generally, one for every switch, two for every cycle) the same values of purity and recovery are found. A situation like the one just described is referred to as *steady-state*.

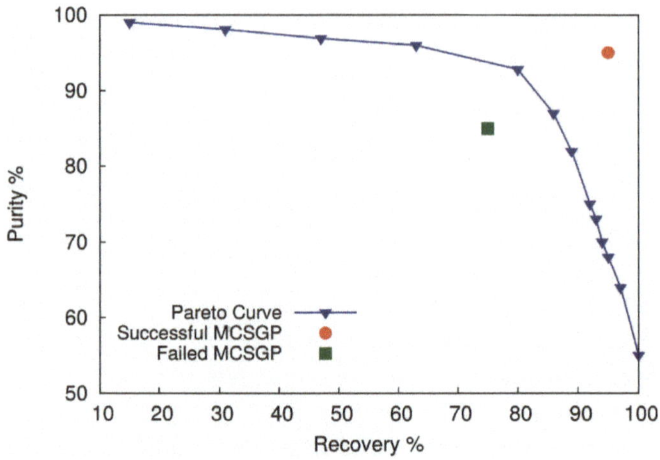


**Fig. 10** Example of a Pareto curve showing the so-called purity-yield trade-off. The red dot and the green square represent the performance of two hypothetical MCSGP processes, as it is explained in the text. *Reproduced with permission from de Luca C, Felletti S, Lievore G, et al: Modern trends in downstream processing of biotherapeutics through continuous chromatography: the potential of multicolumn countercurrent solvent gradient purification,* Trends Analyt Chem *132, 2020b. doi:10.1016/j.trac.2020.116051.*

The set of switching times are the only parameters affecting the comparison between the batch and the continuous performance, because all other parameters are kept constant during the transfer: the amount of feed loaded per volume of stationary phase, the gradient slope, the duration of every step, etc. Anyway, to have a fair comparison between the two processes, a Pareto curve is necessary also for a column with Vcol comparable to the total Vcol of the MCSGP (for instance, it can be twice as long as the MCSGP columns if a twin-column process is considered). The longer column is used as the reference to compare the performance of the processes, being the volume of resin equal.

The pair of values of purity and recovery found at steady-state must be compared to the Pareto curve of the corresponding batch method run on the longer column: two situations can be encountered (see Fig. 10). If the MCSGP point lies below the Pareto curve, the continuous process reaches a lower yield than the batch, at similar purity (green square in Fig. 3), and so the MCSGP process results unsuccessful. On the contrary, the red point lies above the curve when the recovery obtained in continuous conditions is higher than for the batch, meaning when the MCSGP performance overcome that of the batch; so, the continuous process is successful when its point lies in the upper right corner of the diagram. In conclusion, while the Pareto curve of the reference batch (longer column) is needed to compare the performance of the processes, the Pareto curve of the design batch chromatogram (shorter column) is used to set a first trial set of switching times.

If the MCSGP performance is insufficient, the set of characteristic times must be changed. For example, if the pooled product is proven to contain W impurities, it means that $t_C$ should be moved to the left, to recycle the portion of eluent that contaminates the pool and to improve the purity. Otherwise, if the offline analysis of the waste streams draws attention to a too high concentration of the target product in the waste, such as in the S zone, it means that $t_E$ must be moved to the right, to recycle into the system the rear part of the target peak. In general, recovery is affected by times $t_B$ and $t_E$, whereas the purity is influenced on the times defining the product elution window ($t_C$ and $t_D$) (Vogg et al., 2019). The procedure just illustrated does not aim at finding the optimal conditions of a given process, but rather it tries to identify, with very limited experimental effort, conditions satisfying purity constraints.

The pool recovery has a direct impact also on the other performance parameters, especially productivity and, to a lesser extent, solvent consumption. Both from the environmental and the economic point of view, it would be desirable to obtain a higher productivity and a very low solvent consumption, but it must be kept in mind that purity and recovery are the most important parameters for high valuable product, such as therapeutic proteins and peptides, and so they have priority. Sometimes it can happen that MCSGP leads to very good values of recovery but only moderate gains or even small losses in productivity. Nevertheless, these results can be acceptable since it is preferable to focus on the maximization of the recovery when dealing with very expensive bioproducts, to achieve good economic profits. Also, the formula of productivity does not account for the advantages deriving from the automation of the process when scaling it to MCSGP, advantages which are not only economic but also time-related, since continuous processes allow to save the downtimes. Finding the optimal experimental conditions in the process is challenging, and therefore the MCSGP is not always able to outperform the corresponding batch performance (Gerstweiler et al., 2021).

Beside the just described experimental fine-tuning of the working conditions, some authors have also modeled the MCSGP performance, depending on the adsorption isotherms, either linear (Steinebach et al., 2017a; Ströhlein et al., 2006) or nonlinear (Aumann et al., 2007), and the operating conditions, as it will be reported in the next section. Modeling the process is anyway rather complex and sometimes too time-consuming if compared with the experimental fine-tuning.

## 6. Applications of MCSGP

MCSGP finds a wide application range in the purification of high valuable biomolecules where ternary separations are involved. The most successful cases where this continuous technique has been applied concern the separation of protein-based biopharmaceuticals, such as mono-PEGylated proteins, monoclonal antibodies, peptides, but recently it has been exploited also for oligonucleotides and cannabinoids mixtures.

Monoclonal antibodies (mAbs), for instance, are an established class of biotherapeutics: in 2016, more than 50 mAbs had already been approved and 50 were under phase three clinical trials according to FDA, with sales around $75 billion (Ecker et al., 2015; Gjoka et al., 2017; Reichert, 2016). In 2015, Ecker et al. forecasted that, by 2020, 70 or more mAbs would have been present on the market (Ecker et al., 2015); in fact, as of the end of summer 2020 the mAbs market had grown to 125 mAbs approved in Europe or USA (Ecker et al., 2020). The attention toward this class of biomolecules has risen also because of the pandemic situation caused by COVID-19; indeed, after almost 2 years of research, two mAbs (casirivimab and regdanvimab) have been approved as a treatment for infected people who do not require supplemental oxygen (European Medicines Agency, n.d.; Italian Medicines Agency, n.d.). One of the first MCSGP applications developed right after its patent was filed regarded the separation of a mAb from clarified cell culture supernatant (Morbidelli et al., 2007), using three cation exchange columns (three-column MCSGP). They demonstrated that the continuous process led to purities comparable to a batch process performed in affinity chromatography with Protein A, but using much cheaper CEX columns. In the same study, during the separation of three mAbs variants differing only in the number of lysine groups at the C-terminal, MCSGP allowed to increase both the recovery and the purity (93% and 90% respectively), whereas in the batch run the maximum purity achievable at an almost nil recovery (very narrow collection window) was 80%.

Müller-Späth et al. (Müller-Späth et al., 2010) developed a two-step capture process for an immunoglobulin IgG2 (a mAb) purification using MCSGP, also in CEX conditions but with four columns. The MCSGP performance were then compared to the performance of nonaffinity batch run. At a similar yield (around 92–94%) and productivity of 6 and 4 g/L/h respectively, the purity with MCSGP process reached a value greater of 97%, while with the batch it was around 88%. Also, it is worth noting that the MCSGP buffer consumption was half the value obtained for the batch (3.4 vs 6.4 L/g).

In a work by Ulmer et al. (Ulmer et al., 2019), they intended to integrate the upstream and downstream processing of a Fab fragment, deriving from the enzymatic digestion of IgG (upstream). The digested was directly fed into the three-column MCSGP equipment (downstream); this chromatographic step allowed to alleviate the yield-purity trade-off, bringing the yield from 72% to 90% at a purity around 90%.

The separation of the main charge isoform of a mAb from five different isoforms, deriving from Protein A capture, was performed by Steinebach et al. (Steinebach et al., 2017b) both in batch and in twin-column MCSGP, in ion-exchange mode. Particularly, the protein of interest was a 147 kDa human immunoglobulin. The experimental conditions included a NaCl salt gradient, obtained with buffer A: 20 mM phosphate, pH 6.1, and buffer B: 20 mM phosphate, pH 6.1, NaCl 150 mM. As it is usually done, the compensation buffer used for inline dilution was buffer A. For the reference batch, a 5 × 100 mm column was used, whereas for MCSGP two identical columns were used with size 5 × 50 mm, so that the total resin volume was the same, for a fair comparison. Using the strategy described in the previous section to transfer a batch method to continuous technology, it resulted that for a given purity of 92% the yield increased from 85% to 94% with the MCSGP, while the productivity improved from 1.8 to 2.6 g/L/h. The solvent consumption did not show any improvement when scaling the method to MCSGP.

The same separation problem (147 kDa immunoglobulin) was also exploited by Vogg and coworkers (Vogg et al., 2019) to characterize the twin-column MCSGP process with respect to the set of switching times, that represent its only degrees of freedom. It turned out that purity is influenced by the times defining the collection windows, and the presence of weak or strong impurities must be attributed to the beginning and the end of the pooling step respectively. On the other hand, recovery is influenced basically by $t_B$ and $t_E$.

Beside mAbs, other classes of amino acid-containing molecules have been purified by MCSGP, such as other kinds of proteins and peptides. A mixture of proteins showing different degrees of PEGylation was separated through anion exchange chromatography in order to isolate the mono-PEGylated variant (alpha-Lactalbumin). Higher yield and productivity were obtained (Subramanian, 2005).

Recently, Kim and coworkers (Kim et al., 2021) separated a PEG-protein conjugate (PEGylated lysozyme) with MCSGP, using a strong cation exchange resin. The mobile phases included sodium phosphate as equilibration buffer and sodium chloride as elution buffer. They managed to obtain an increase in yield of about 17%, whereas the productivity was substantially unchanged, at a purity specification of 80%.

Considering peptides, the first one to be purified by means of three- or six-column MCSGP was calcitonin, in 2007 (Aumann and Morbidelli, 2007, 2008; Aumann et al., 2007). Reversed-phase conditions and a gradient of acetonitrile have been used. At a target purity of 93%, MCSGP managed to achieve a recovery around 100%, compared to a maximum value equal to 66% obtained for the batch. This gain, nevertheless, did not reflect in an improvement in productivity. The process performance has also been simulated through a chromatographic lumped kinetic model, keeping into account the strong nonlinear competitive bi-Langmuir isotherm of calcitonin. The model allows to understand the effect of different operating conditions (feed flow rate, switching times, etc.) on the performance (Aumann et al., 2007).

A comparison between batch and MCSGP processes for the purification of an unspecified peptide has been described by Müller-Späth et al. (Müller-Späth et al., 2013). At a final purity of around 99%, yield was improved by 4 times, and productivity by 10 times, while the solvent consumption decreased by 70% (from 3.5 to 1 L of solvent per gram of purified product) using three-column MCSGP in reversed-phase conditions.

Another polypeptide purified in reversed-phase conditions by means of three-column MCSGP led to improvements both in productivity and in solvent consumption: the first one increased by 25 times whereas the second one was reduced by 60% (Aumann et al., 2009). For a particularly challenging polypeptide, it was even demonstrated through a process modeling formerly developed that the MCSGP process led to a solvent consumption of only 8 L/g, which corresponded to a 10-fold decrease if compared to the typical case of batch process with ideal manual recycling (Morbidelli et al., 2007).

The authors of this chapter, together with coworkers, have also investigated the feasibility of the MCSGP purification on two peptide crude mixtures synthesized industrially. Particularly, glucagon is a 29 amino acids peptide which has been separated in reversed-phase conditions, using mobile phases containing an ammonium acetate buffer and acetonitrile and a $C_8$ stationary phase, packed in one column 250 × 4.6 mm (batch) and two columns 150 × 4.6 mm (for the MCSGP). It resulted that, at a comparable purity around 89%, MCSGP could bring an increase of +23% in the recovery, even if to the detriment of productivity, because in MCSGP, during the interconnected steps, very low flow rates are used, which lengthen the duration of the process. However, as already said above, in case of very expensive product it is preferable to save as much target product as possible, and an increase in the recovery can compensate the loss in productivity. The experimental conditions reported in the article, moreover, were not intended to be the optimal ones (de Luca et al., 2020a).

The second peptide considered is icatibant, a small peptidomimetics made of 10 amino acids, which was separated in reversed-phase chromatography as well, with triethylamine phosphate buffer and acetonitrile. The $C_{18}$ columns dimensions were 250 × 4.6 mm for the reference batch and 150 × 4.6 for the twin columns in MCSGP. In this particular case, the performance obtained with the continuous process significantly overcame the batch, at a purity greater than 99%. The recovery increased by almost seven times (from 12% to 95%), and the productivity improved by six times (from 1.13 to 7.65 g/L/h). Because of these improvements, the solvent consumption decreased by 80%, a remarkable result also from the point of view of the environmental impact (de Luca et al., 2021a).

Besides the already mentioned proteinaceous mixtures, MCSGP has lately proven to be effective also in the purification of other kinds of biomolecules. Chromacon AG—A YMC Company, the company producing the ContiChrom CUBE, the main equipment where the MCSGP process can be performed, has released two application notes regarding the purification of cannabinoids and oligonucleotides mixtures through MCSGP. Cannabinoids are currently under investigation for their therapeutic properties, whereas oligonucleotides are emerging as a class of promising therapeutic drugs, thanks to their ability to specifically regulate gene expression. In the first case, MCSGP has been successfully used to remove the psychoactive tetrahydrocannabinol (THC) from a cannabinoids hemp extract, to obtain a THC-free product (ChromaCon—A YMC Company, 2019a). In the second case, the continuous process allowed to double the mass recovered, at a target purity of 92% (Catani et al., 2020; ChromaCon—A YMC Company, 2019b). Recently, Weldon et al. used also MSCGP to purify, in reversed-phase chromatography, a *N*-acetylgalactosamine (GalNAc)-cluster-conjugated DNA-LNA gapmer oligonucleotide, increasing yield from 52% to 91%, at 94% purity. Similar values of productivity and buffer consumption were found for the batch and the MCSGP (Weldon et al., 2021).

As it can be noted from all the cited examples, MCSGP becomes particularly appealing and successful in case of difficult and tricky ternary separations of costly biomolecules with therapeutic applications, exhibiting a steep yield-purity trade-off curve.

## 7. Conclusions

In the last decades, great attention has been paid to the manufacturing of biopharmaceuticals. Remarkable improvements have been brought to upstream techniques, but they have not been followed by similar technological developments in the downstream processing. The purifications steps, often performed through chromatographic techniques, are still the bottleneck in the production of biomolecules, because they are time-consuming during the development phases and expensive, even in terms of materials and solvents. Also, during these steps, the strict purity requirements must be compulsorily met, which is a hard task due to the presence of critical product-related impurities.

In this frame, continuous chromatographic techniques are rapidly gaining importance as promising candidates for the intensification of downstream processing of biomolecules with therapeutic scopes, such as proteins and peptides. MCSGP is particularly appealing because of its intrinsic features, including the possibility to use a linear solvent gradient, the internal recycling of the impure side fractions and the automation of the process, that allow to outperform the single-column (batch) chromatography. Therefore, the performance of the batch, especially in terms of recovery, but sometimes also in terms of productivity and solvent consumption, can be overcome with this continuous or semicontinuous process, alleviating the yield-purity trade-off typical of batch processes. These improvements involve significant cost savings on industrial scale and, what's more, can contribute to reduce the environmental impact of the manufacturing, when it is possible to reduce solvent consumption. Moreover, this technology employs traditional hardware (pumps, valves, etc.) and this could make MCSGP a more easily scalable process.

MCSGP has proven to be suitable, at laboratory and pilot scale, for difficult purifications of different classes of biomolecules, including proteins, mAbs, peptides, but also oligonucleotides and cannabinoids, as demonstrated by the rich literature reported. The good preliminary results and study conducted until now suggest that the establishment of this technology at all production scales can be envisaged, even for further applications in the field of biomolecules.

## References


Aumann L, Morbidelli M: *Method and device for chromatographic purification. EP1877769B1*, 2006.

Aumann L, Morbidelli M: A continuous multicolumn countercurrent solvent gradient purification (MCSGP) process, *Biotechnol Bioeng* 98:1043–1055, 2007. https://doi.org/10.1002/BIT.21527.

Aumann L, Morbidelli M: A semicontinuous 3-column countercurrent solvent gradient purification (MCSGP) process, *Biotechnol Bioeng* 99:728–733, 2008. https://doi.org/10.1002/bit.21585.

Aumann L, Stroehlein G, Morbidelli M: Parametric study of a 6-column countercurrent solvent gradient purification (MCSGP) unit, *Biotechnol Bioeng* 98:1029–1042, 2007. https://doi.org/10.1002/BIT.21529.

Aumann L, Morbidelli M, Schenkel B, Stroehlein G: Protein peptide purification using the multicolumn countercurrent solvent gradient purification (MCSGP), *Biopharm Int* 22, 2009.

Baur D, Angarita M, Müller-Späth T, Steinebach F, Morbidelli M: Comparison of batch and continuous multi-column protein A capture processes by optimal design, *Biotechnol J* 11:920–931, 2016. https://doi.org/10.1002/biot.201500481.

Burnouf T, Radosevich M: Affinity chromatography in the industrial purification of plasma proteins for therapeutic use, *J Biochem Biophys Methods* 49:575–586, 2001. https://doi.org/10.1016/S0165-022X(01)00221-4.

Carter PJ: Introduction to current and future protein therapeutics: a protein engineering perspective, *Exp Cell Res* 317:1261–1269, 2011. https://doi.org/10.1016/J.YEXCR.2011.02.013.

Catani M, de Luca C, Medeiros Garcia Alcântara J, et al.: Oligonucleotides: current trends and innovative applications in the synthesis, characterization, and purification, *Biotechnol J* 15, 2020. https://doi.org/10.1002/biot.201900226.

Chibério AS, Policarpo GFM, Antunes JC, Santos TP, Ribeiro RPPL, Mota JPB: Batch chromatography with recycle lag. II—Physical realization and experimental validation, *J Chromatogr A* 1623:461211, 2020. https://doi.org/10.1016/J.CHROMA.2020.461211.

ChromaCon—A YMC Company: *Highly pure cannabidiol (CBD) by twin-column chromatography (MCSGP)*, 2019a.

ChromaCon—A YMC Company: *Purification of a therapeutic oligonucleotide using twin-column chromatography (MCSGP)*, 2019b.

Curling J: The development of antibody purification technologies, In *Process scale purification of antibodies*, Hoboken, NJ, USA, 2008, John Wiley & Sons, Inc., pp 25–52. https://doi.org/10.1002/9780470444894.ch2.

de Luca C, Felletti S, Lievore G, et al.: From batch to continuous chromatographic purification of a therapeutic peptide through multicolumn countercurrent solvent gradient purification, *J Chromatogr A* 1625, 2020a. https://doi.org/10.1016/j.chroma.2020.461304.

de Luca C, Felletti S, Lievore G, et al.: Modern trends in downstream processing of biotherapeutics through continuous chromatography: the potential of multicolumn countercurrent solvent gradient purification, *Trends Analyt Chem* 132, 2020b. https://doi.org/10.1016/j.trac.2020.116051.

de Luca C, Felletti S, Bozza D, et al.: Process intensification for the purification of peptidomimetics: the case of icatibant through multicolumn countercurrent solvent gradient purification (MCSGP), *Ind Eng Chem Res* 60:6826–6834, 2021a. https://doi.org/10.1021/acs.iecr.1c00520.

de Luca C, Lievore G, Bozza D, et al.: Downstream processing of therapeutic peptides by means of preparative liquid chromatography, *Molecules* 26, 2021b. https://doi.org/10.3390/molecules26154688.

Dimitrov DS: Therapeutic proteins, *Methods Mol Biol* 899:1–26, 2012. https://doi.org/10.1007/978-1-61779-921-1_1.

Ecker DM, Dana Jones S, Levine HL: The therapeutic monoclonal antibody market, *MAbs* 7:9–14, 2015. https://doi.org/10.4161/19420862.2015.989042.

Ecker DM, Crawford TJ, Seymour P: The therapeutic monoclonal antibody product market, *Bioprocess Int*, 2020.

European Medicines Agency COVID-19: EMA recommends authorisation of two monoclonal antibody medicines n.d. https://www.ema.europa.eu/en/news/covid-19-ema-recommends-authorisation-two-monoclonal-antibody-medicines (accessed December 22, 2021).

Gerstweiler L, Bi J, Middelberg APJ: Continuous downstream bioprocessing for intensified manufacture of biopharmaceuticals and antibodies, *Chem Eng Sci* 231:116272, 2021. https://doi.org/10.1016/J.CES.2020.116272.

Girard V, Hilbold NJ, Ng CKS, et al.: Large-scale monoclonal antibody purification by continuous chromatography, from process design to scale-up, *J Biotechnol* 213:65–73, 2015. https://doi.org/10.1016/J.JBIOTEC.2015.04.026.

Gjoka X, Gantier R, Schofield M: Transfer of a three step mAb chromatography process from batch to continuous: optimizing productivity to minimize consumable requirements, *J Biotechnol* 242:11–18, 2017. https://doi.org/10.1016/J.JBIOTEC.2016.12.005.

Grossmann C, Ströhlein G, Morari M, Morbidelli M: Optimizing model predictive control of the chromatographic multi-column solvent gradient purification (MCSGP) process, *J Process Control* 20:618–629, 2010. https://doi.org/10.1016/J.JPROCONT.2010.02.013.

Hober S, Nord K, Linhult M: Protein a chromatography for antibody purification, *J Chromatogr B* 848:40–47, 2007. https://doi.org/10.1016/J.JCHROMB.2006.09.030.

Houp RC: Ultrafiltration and diafiltration, *J Valid Technol*, 2009.

Italian Medicines Agency Uso degli anticorpi monoclonali per COVID-19 n.d. https://www.aifa.gov.it/en/web/guest/uso-degli-anticorpi-monoclonali (accessed December 22, 2021).

Kim TK, Botti C, Angelo J, et al.: Experimental design of the multicolumn countercurrent solvent gradient purification (MCSGP) unit for the separation of PEGylated proteins, *Ind Eng Chem Res* 60:10764–10776, 2021. https://doi.org/10.1021/ACS.IECR.1C01345/SUPPL_FILE/IE1C01345_SI_001.PDF.

Knäblein J, editor: *Modern biopharmaceuticals: recent success stories*, 2013, Wiley-VCH Verlag. https://doi.org/10.1002/9783527669417.

Krättli M, Müller-Späth T, Morbidelli M: Multifraction separation in countercurrent chromatography (MCSGP), *Biotechnol Bioeng* 110:2436–2444, 2013. https://doi.org/10.1002/BIT.24901.

Leader B, Baca QJ, Golan DE: Protein therapeutics: a summary and pharmacological classification, *Nat Rev Drug Discov* 7(1):21–39, 2008. https://doi.org/10.1038/nrd2399.

Liu HF, Ma J, Winter C, Bayer R: Recovery and purification process development for monoclonal antibody production, *MAbs* 2:480–499, 2010. https://doi.org/10.4161/mabs.2.5.12645.
Mazzotti M, Storti G, Morbidelli M: Optimal operation of simulated moving bed units for nonlinear chromatographic separations, *J Chromatogr A* 769:3–24, 1997. https://doi.org/10.1016/S0021-9673(97)00048-4.
Morbidelli M, Müller-Späth T, Tarafder A, Stroehlein G, Aumann L: Continuous processing: the multicolumn countercurrent solvent gradient purification process, *Biopharm Int*, 2007.
Müller-Späth T, Morbidelli M: Multicolumn countercurrent gradient chromatography for the purification of biopharmaceuticals, In *Continuous processing in pharmaceutical manufacturing*, 2015, pp 227–254. https://doi.org/10.1002/9783527673681.CH10.
Müller-Späth T, Aumann L, Ströhlein G, et al.: Two step capture and purification of IgG2 using multicolumn countercurrent solvent gradient purification (MCSGP), *Biotechnol Bioeng* 107:974–984, 2010. https://doi.org/10.1002/BIT.22887.
Müller-Späth T, Ströhlein G, Lyngberg O, Maclean D: Enabling high purities and yields in therapeutic peptide purification using multicolumn countercurrent solvent gradient purification, *Chim Oggi Chem Today* 31:56–60, 2013.
Pfister D, Nicoud L, Morbidelli M: *Continuous biopharmaceutical processes: chromatography, bioconjugation, and protein stability*, 2018, Cambridge University Press. https://doi.org/10.1017/9781108332897.
Reichert JM: Antibodies to watch in 2016, *MAbs* 8:197–204, 2016. https://doi.org/10.1080/19420862.2015.1125583.
Remington KM: Fundamental strategies for viral clearance, *Bioprocess Int*, 2015.
Schramm H, Kaspereit M, Kienle A, Seidel-Morgenstern A: Simulated moving bed process with cyclic modulation of the feed concentration, *J Chromatogr A* 1006:77–86, 2003. https://doi.org/10.1016/S0021-9673(03)00327-3.
Segovia-Hernández JG, Bonilla-Petriciolet A: *Process intensification in chemical engineering: design, optimization and control*, 2016, Springer International Publishing. https://doi.org/10.1007/978-3-319-28392-0.
Steinebach F, Krättli M, Storti G, Morbidelli M: Equilibrium theory based design space for the multicolumn countercurrent solvent gradient purification process, *Ind Eng Chem Res* 56:13482–13489, 2017a. https://doi.org/10.1021/acs.iecr.7b00569.
Steinebach F, Ulmer N, Decker L, Aumann L, Morbidelli M: Experimental design of a twin-column countercurrent gradient purification process, *J Chromatogr A* 1492:19–26, 2017b. https://doi.org/10.1016/j.chroma.2017.02.049.
Ströhlein G, Aumann L, Mazzotti M, Morbidelli M: A continuous, counter-current multi-column chromatographic process incorporating modifier gradients for ternary separations, *J Chromatogr A* 1126:338–346, 2006. https://doi.org/10.1016/j.chroma.2006.05.011.
Subramanian G: *Continuous processing in pharmaceutical manufacturing*, 2005.
Tarafder A, Aumann L, Morbidelli M: The role of ion-pairing in peak deformations in overloaded reversed-phase chromatography of peptides, *J Chromatogr A* 1217:7065–7073, 2010. https://doi.org/10.1016/j.chroma.2010.09.007.
Ulmer N, Ristanovic D, Morbidelli M: Process for continuous fab production by digestion of IgG, *Biotechnol J* 14:1800677, 2019. https://doi.org/10.1002/BIOT.201800677.
Vogg S, Ulmer N, Souquet J, Broly H, Morbidelli M: Experimental evaluation of the impact of intrinsic process parameters on the performance of a continuous chromatographic polishing unit (MCSGP), *Biotechnol J* 14, 2019. https://doi.org/10.1002/biot.201800732.
Walsh G: Biopharmaceutical benchmarks 2018, *Nat Biotechnol* 36:1136–1145, 2018. https://doi.org/10.1038/NBT.4305.

Warikoo V, Godawat R, Brower K, et al.: Integrated continuous production of recombinant therapeutic proteins, *Biotechnol Bioeng* 109:3018–3029, 2012. https://doi.org/10.1002/BIT.24584.

Weldon R, Lill J, Olbrich M, Schmidt P, Müller-Späth T: Purification of a GalNAc-cluster-conjugated oligonucleotide by reversed-phase twin-column continuous chromatography, *J Chromatogr A* 462734, 2021. https://doi.org/10.1016/J.CHROMA.2021.462734.

Yin L, Chen X, Vicini P, Rup B, Hickling TP: Therapeutic outcomes, assessments, risk factors and mitigation efforts of immunogenicity of therapeutic protein products, *Cell Immunol* 295:118–126, 2015. https://doi.org/10.1016/J.CELLIMM.2015.03.002.

Zapadka KL, Becher FJ, Gomes dos Santos AL, Jackson SE: Factors affecting the physical stability (aggregation) of peptide therapeutics, *Interface Focus* 7, 2017. https://doi.org/10.1098/rsfs.2017.0030.

CHAPTER FOUR

# Potential of fluidized bed adsorption technology in continuous bioproduct recovery and purification

**Lisa-Marie Herlevi**[a] **and Hector Marcelo Fernandez Lahore**[a,b,*]
[a]Jacobs University Bremen, Bremen, Germany
[b]Luxembourg Institute of Science and Technology, Belvaux, Luxembourg
*Corresponding author: e-mail address: m.fernandez-lahore@jacobs-university.de

## Contents



## Abstract

Fluidized bed adsorption is less commonly applied for purification of proteins although offering advantages over packed bed chromatography by having increased voidage in the bed allowing particulate matter to pass through the column. Conventional downstream processing scheme can be intensified by combining clarification and primary capture into one stage with the help of fluidized or expanded bed adsorption (EBA). Adsorbents applied for fluidized bed systems require specific considerations for particle size and density affecting the quality of fluidization. Additionally, biomass-adsorbent interactions are an important factor influencing the adsorption and fluidization properties, and with the help of surface energetics they can be quantified, and various approaches have been taken to mitigate this phenomena. In the attempts of shifting bioprocessing industry into continuous manufacturing new chromatographic

*Advances in Chemical Engineering*, Volume 59
ISSN 0065-2377
https://doi.org/10.1016/bs.ache.2022.03.006

technologies based on packed bed technology such as simulated moving bed (SMB) and periodic counter current (PCC) chromatography have emerged. Continuous chromatography with fluidized bed technology has been established by having both process streams and resin in continuous motion and with further efforts into technology development could offer an alternative to SMB and PCC.

## 1. Introduction

Contrasted with packed bed chromatography, liquid-solid fluidized bed technology can be employed for purification of proteins from unclarified feedstock due to increased voidage of the bed allowing particulate matter to flow through the column without leading to significant increase in pressure drop throughout the bed (Chase, 1994). The first steps of downstream processing, usually including centrifugation and membrane filtration, result in broth volume reduction and some purification, while leading to long processing time and significant losses in yield (Harrison et al., 2003; Elmar et al., 2006; Hubbuch et al., n.d.). Therefore, liquid-solid fluidized bed technology can potentially be applied as an integrative step for downstream processing combining clarification, primary capture and concentration, and hence minimizing the number of required unit operations (Fig. 1).

## 2. Liquid-solid fluidized bed technology

Expanded bed adsorption (EBA) is a relatively new chromatographic technique that differs from conventional liquid-solid fluidized bed technology in terms of degree of mixing. The first examples of EBA were published by Chase and Draeger (Chase, 1994; Chase and Draeger, 1992a,b) three decades ago, and since then the technology has been commercialized and extensively studied as an integrative step for purification of biologics ranging from industrial enzymes (da Silva Padilha et al., 2009; Pessoa et al., 1996; Silvino Dos Santos et al., 2002) to high value monoclonal antibodies (Thömmes et al., 1996; Thömmes et al., 1995a, 1995b). Magnetically stabilized fluidized beds (MSFB) have the characteristics of expanded bed, low back-mixing and plug flow liquid motion, which are achieved by applying uniform magnetic field to stabilize magnetically susceptible particles (Chetty and Burns, 1991; Tong and Sun, 2003). Despite the potential application of MSFB as an alternative for packed bed chromatography, inexpensive magnetic carriers and separators are needed for large scale

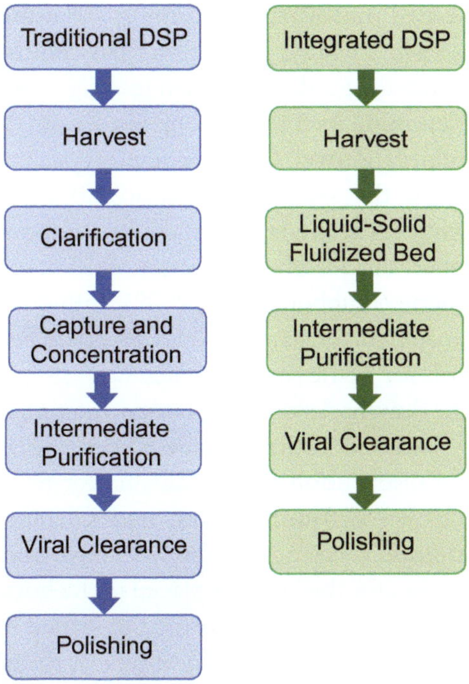


**Fig. 1** Process flow sheet comparison between a traditional downstream process (DSP) and an integrated approach. *Adapted from D'Souza RN, Azevedo AM, Aires-Barros MR, et al: Emerging technologies for the integration and intensification of downstream bioprocesses.* Pharm Bioprocess, *1:423–440, 2013.*

application (Safarik and Safarikova, 2004). Further disadvantages include heat generation when producing the electromagnetic field, and instability of ferromagnetic particles in sodium hydroxide, which is a common cleaning agent used in downstream processing (Chase, 1994).

## 2.1 Expanded bed adsorption

A characteristic feature of EBA that differentiates the process from a conventional liquid-solid fluidized bed technology, used in the chemical industry since the early 1920s, is the particle size distribution forming a classified bed where larger adsorbent particles are found from the bottom of the expanded bed and smaller from the top part of the bed, resulting in lower back-mixing, and ideally leads to a plug-flow profile through the column (Hubbuch et al., n.d.; Hjorth, 1997; Shukla et al., 2007). The main difference between packed bed and expanded bed column is in the flow distribution system that ensures an even distribution of the flow over the cross-section of the bed, necessary for forming a classified bed (Hubbuch et al., n.d.; Chase, 1994). The first generation EBA columns used perforated plates and metal meshes for fluid distribution leading to issues with aggregation and required cleaning before elution, hindering the application for pharmaceutical products (Zuwei, 2015). Therefore, a rotating fluid distributor was designed for the second generation EBA columns leading to increased back-mixing in the lower part of the bed, although due to absence of bottom net to retain the adsorbent particles, elution could be performed only in expanded mode (Hubbuch et al., 2002). Influence of different fluid distribution systems on hydrodynamic properties of the bed will be discussed further in the section for bed hydrodynamics.

To overcome the drawbacks related to second generation EBA columns, Chang and Chang designed a stirred fluidized bed (SFB) column adapted with a rotating fluid distribution system suitable for feedstocks containing large sized particulates (>70 μm) (Chang and Chang, 2006; Hubbuch et al., 2002). The crude feedstock is applied above the distributor plate and support net and inlet for the buffer is placed in the bottom of the column (Fig. 2), allowing the elution to be performed in settled bed mode without leading to problems with net clogging. Additionally, the SFB column could achieve a well-mixed zone at the bottom of the column at a lower rotating speed of the agitator (approximately 100 rpm) in comparison to UpFront

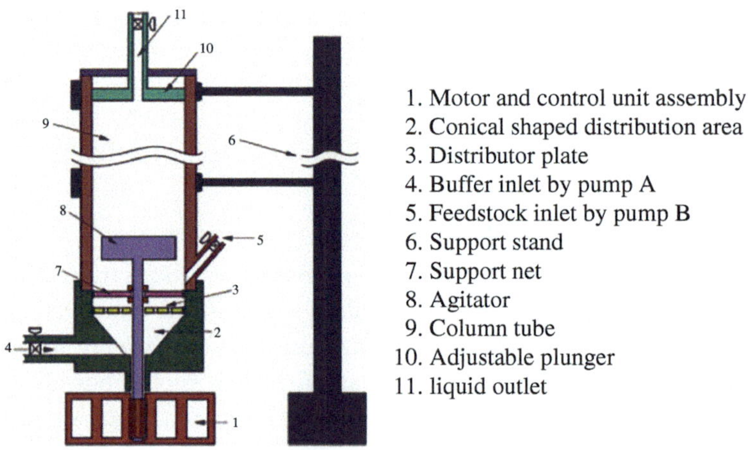


**Fig. 2** Schematic of stirred fluidized bed column. *Adapted from Chang Y, Chang I: Method development for direct recovery of lysozyme from highly crude chicken egg white by stirred fluidized bed technique.* Biochem Eng J, *30(1):63–75, 2006. doi:10.1016/j.bej.2006.02.006.*

EBA column equipped with paddle agitator (approximately 300 rpm). During the capture step, both feedstock and buffer are pumped into the column (Chang and Chang, 2006).

The SFB column has been successfully applied for direct purification of lysozyme from crude chicken egg white (CEW) with recovery yields above 90% and purification factor yielding up to 40 folds, outperforming the traditional purification techniques involving pre-treatment of CEW (Chang and Chang, 2006; Chen et al., 2019; Show et al., 2021). Other examples of direct protein recovery from unclarified feedstock with SFB system include purification of malate dehydrogenase with a yield of 73.6% and a purification factor of 73.5 (Chen et al., 2018), and recombinant enhanced green fluorescent protein with a yield between 95% and 98% and a purification factor of 3 folds (Song et al., 2020). Despite the advantages of SFB system, its application hasn't been nearly as extensively reported in comparison to EBA.

The operation and optimization of each stage for capture and purification employing EBA are similar to a packed bed column which consists of equilibrium and dynamic capacity studies. In a batch-wise operation the first stage starts by expanding the settled bed by applying an upward flow from bottom of the column until a stable expanded bed, approximately twice its settled height, and equilibration are achieved (Fig. 3). To avoid further expansion of the bed, the flow velocity needs to be lowered due to physical properties of the feedstock, namely viscosity. Depending on the fluid distribution system, subsequent washing and elution stages can be performed in expanded or packed mode, by settling the bed, and using either a downward or upward flow. A cleaning-in-place (CIP) procedure is followed by the elution to ensure removal of all impurities and to prevent carryover of material between batches, and to maintain the functionality of the adsorbent (Chang and Chase, 1996; Chase, 1994; Hjorth, 1997).

The choice of operational flow velocity is made to achieve high capacity for the target product and good chromatography resolution which are influenced by physical and chemical properties of the adsorbent and feedstock. The operating parameters have more influence on adsorption performance and bed stability when processing unclarified feedstocks, and need to be additionally studied when developing a purification protocol (Chang and Chase, 1996) The scaling-up procedure for EBA is performed by maintaining the column length and linear flow velocity constant while increasing the column diameter, and the parameters used for verification include degree of bed expansion, degree of mixing of liquid phase and breakthrough capacity (Bermejo et al., 2007; Frej et al., 1997).

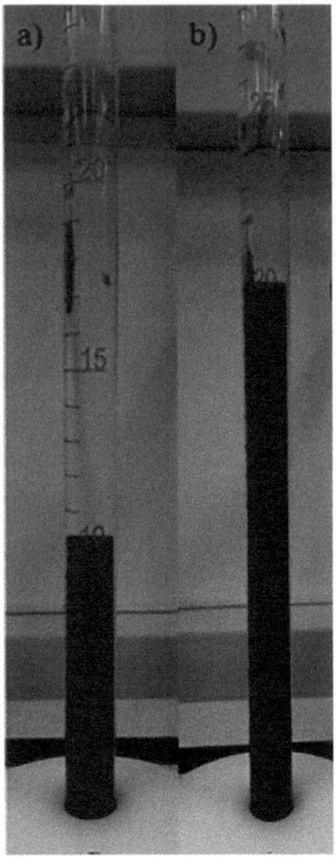


**Fig. 3** Expanded bed adsorption column operation: (A) settled bed and (B) fluidized bed.

## 2.2 Adsorbent materials

Preliminary work carried out in the early 1990s used conventional chromatographic adsorbents for packed bed applications manufactured from cross-linked agarose to create a stable expanded bed. However, to achieve sufficient degree of bed expansion, inconveniently low linear-flow velocities were required (10–30 $cm\,h^{-1}$), and therefore adsorbents designed specifically for fluidized bed applications were needed (Chase, 1994). High flow velocity, needed for the best productivity, and highly viscous feedstock require an adsorbent with an increased size or density, achieved either by using a high-density porous material such as commercial Relisorb adsorbent manufactured from a polymethacrylate polymer or by combining a non-porous heavy material with a porous lighter material, such as commercial Streamline adsorbents incorporating small quartz particles in agarose beads (Fig. 4) (Hubbuch et al., n.d.; Chase, 1994; Pålsson et al., 2000).

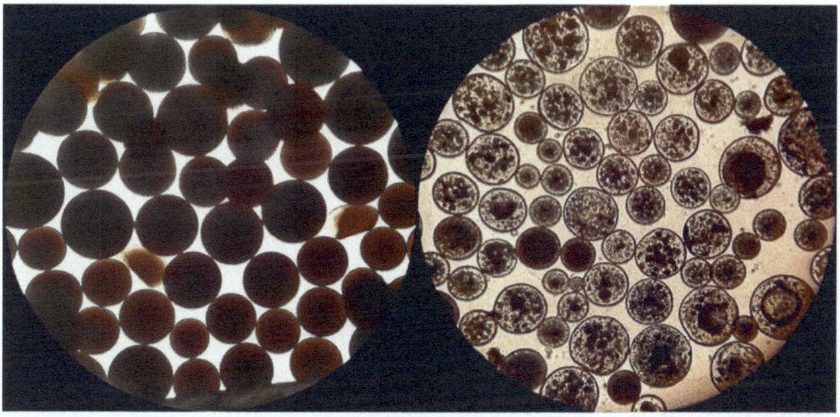

**Fig. 4** Strategies for expanded bed adsorbent design: (A) polymeric material and (B) densified agarose.

**Table 1** Commercially available expanded bed adsorbents.

| Adsorbent (manufacturer) | Base material | Densifier | Size (μm) | Density (mg/mL) | Reference |
|---|---|---|---|---|---|
| Streamline™ (Cytiva) | Agarose | Quartz | 100–300 | 1.2 | a |
| Rhobust® (Upfront Chromatography) | Agarose | Tungsten carbide | 20–300 | 2.5–3.5 | b |
| Relisorb™ (Resindion) | Polymethacrylate | – | 200–500 | 1.1 | c |

[a]https://www.cytivalifesciences.com
[b]https://www.upfront-dk.com
[c]https://www.resindion.com

Commercially available adsorbents for EBA and their physical properties are listed in Table 1. Agarose is the most extensively studied adsorbent material for EBA, and densifiers incorporated with it include glass (Zhou et al., 2007), nickel (Asghari et al., 2012; Rezvani et al., 2014), zinc (Asghari et al., 2012), and zirconia-silica (Jahanshahi et al., 2003). Other polysaccharides that have been explored as an adsorbent material are agar-agar (Asgari et al., 2014), cellulose (Lei et al., 2005; Lin et al., 2006; Xia et al., 2008), and carrageenan (Abatari et al., 2017; Mohsenkhani et al., 2015).

Wright et al. studied the effects of feedstock viscosity and degree of bed expansion on adsorption performance of adsorbents with a macroporous structure and ceramic backbone filled with a hydrogel. In general, intraparticle mass transfer resistance was more significant than increased axial dispersion under all conditions. However, the adsorbent with a ceramic backbone could maintain its performance under high degrees of bed expansion due to hyper-diffusive adsorption property unlike the macroporous structure that suffered from intraparticle diffusion limitations. For the hydrogel filled ceramic adsorbent, film mass transfer effects were more significant with increased feedstock viscosity. In addition to the structure of the adsorbent, pore diffusion, film mass transport and dispersion are also influenced by the diameter of the adsorbent particles, making it a crucial parameter for adsorbent design. Intraparticle mass transfer resistance can be reduced by minimizing the particle diameter achieved for example by using a pellicular matrix with an inert core and a porous surface layer, which leads to decreased diffusion distance, and consequently leads to increased breakthrough capacity (Karau et al., 1997; Pålsson et al., 2000).

## 2.3 Bed hydrodynamics

An important method for characterization of liquid-solid fluidized bed is the Richardson-Zaki (RZ) correlation which predicts linear superficial fluid velocity necessary to achieve a desired bed expansion by using terminal settling velocity of the particles, $U_t$, voidage of the bed, $\varepsilon$, and expansion index or Richardson-Zaki coefficient, n, as shown in Eq. (1) (Richardson and Zaki, 1954):

$$U = U_t \cdot \varepsilon^n \tag{1}$$

Theoretical terminal settling velocity is determined by Stokes law from Eq. (2):

$$U_t = \frac{(\rho_p - \rho_l) d_p^2 g}{18\eta} \tag{2}$$

where $d_p$ is the particle diameter, $\rho_p$ is the density of the particle, and $\rho_l$ is the density of the liquid, and $\eta$ is the viscosity of the liquid phase. The voidage of the bed is calculated from Eq. 3 (Thömmes et al., 1996) where $\varepsilon_0$ is the void fraction of sedimented bed, and $H_0$ and $H$ stand for the settled bed and expanded bed height, respectively. $\varepsilon$ is determined experimentally by measuring $H$ at various fluid velocities. $\varepsilon_0$ can be assumed to be 0.4 which is confirmed by Willoughby et al. (Thömmes et al., 1996; Willoughby et al., 2000).

$$\varepsilon = 1 - (1 - \varepsilon_0)\frac{H_0}{H} \tag{3}$$

n and $U_t$ for any fluid velocity can be obtained from linear regression of ln $U$ vs. ln$\varepsilon$ as shown in Eq. (4):

$$lnU = ln\,U_t + nln\varepsilon \tag{4}$$

Fig. 5 demonstrates how the commercial expanded bed adsorbents from Table 1 differentiate from each other by the degree of bed expansion, $E = \frac{H}{H_0}$, determined experimentally in UpFront FastLine 10 column (Upfront Chromatography, Denmark) connected to ÄKTA FPLC system.

Among the tested adsorbents, the Rhobust adsorbent with a highest density and smallest average particle size, and the Relisorb adsorbent with a largest average particle size and lowest density, could tolerate high linear velocities better in comparison to the Streamline adsorbent, which experienced more significant bed expansion under moderate flow rates. This behavior is correlated with the Richardson-Zaki index obtained from the

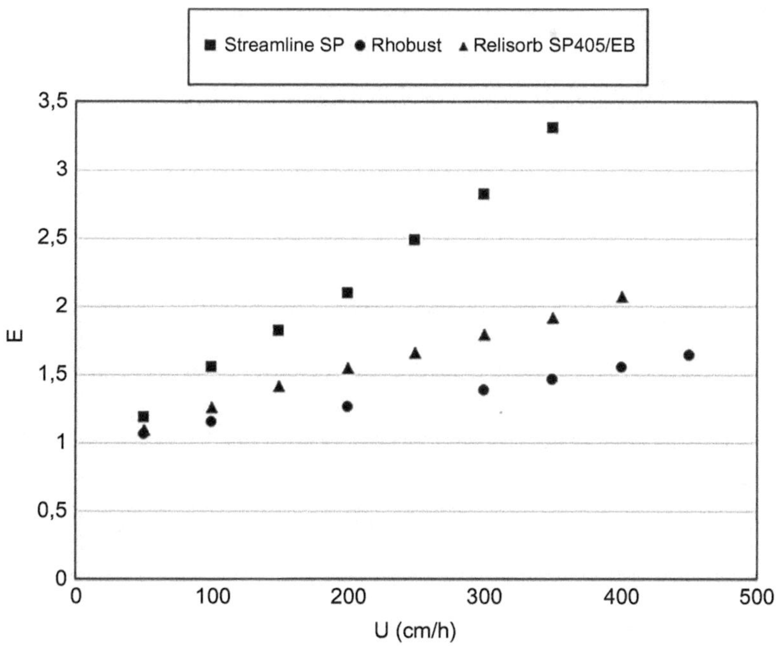


**Fig. 5** Expansion ratios of commercial expanded bed adsorbents: Streamline SP (■), Rhobust (●), and Relisorb SP405/EB (▲).

**Table 2** Richardson-Zaki index for commercial expanded bed adsorbents.

| **Adsorbent** | **n** |
|---|---|
| Streamline SP | 4.16 |
| Rhobust | 5.94 |
| Relisorb SP405/EB | 4.66 |

experimental data presented I Table 2, and showing that increase of the value corresponds to increased resistance to bed expansion.

Mixing of a liquid phase in a fluidized bed is predominantly influenced by the ratio of bed height to diameter of the column, $\frac{H}{d}$, and linear fluid velocity (Thömmes et al., 1995a, 1995b). Degree of axial mixing can be calculated from dimensionless Bodenstein number, $Bo$, that describes the ratio of convective to diffusional mass transport

$$Bo = \frac{uH}{D_{ax}} \tag{5}$$

where $u$ stands for the linear flow velocity, $H$ the height of the bed, and $D_{ax}$ the axial mixing coefficient. The value of $Bo$ can be experimentally measured by residence time distribution (RTD) studies by applying a pulse of tracer such as acetone, to calculate the RTD function as

$$E(t) = \frac{C(t)}{\int_0^\infty C(t)dt} \tag{6}$$

where $C$ is the concentration of the tracer. The variance which represents the square of the distribution when passing the column exit is calculated as

$$\sigma^2 = \int_0^\infty (t - \bar{t})^2 E(t)dt = \mu_2 - \mu_1^2 \tag{7}$$

where $\mu_1$ and $\mu_2$ are the first and second moment, respectively, defined as

$$\mu_1 = \frac{\sum_i t_i C_i \Delta t_i}{\sum_i C_i \Delta t_i} \tag{8}$$

$$\mu_2 = \frac{\sum_i t_i^2 C_i \Delta t_i}{\sum_i C_i \Delta t_i} \tag{9}$$

and by describing the fluidized bed as an open vessel, *Bo* can be calculated from the dimensionless variance according to Eq. (11) (Levenspiel, 1999).

$$\sigma_\theta^2 = \frac{\sigma^2}{\mu_1} = \frac{2}{Bo} + \frac{8}{Bo^2} \tag{10}$$

Since the adsorption capacity of liquid-solid fluidized bed is affected by the hydrodynamic properties, axial mixing should be minimized by increasing the value of *Bo* number, either by increasing the ratio of $\frac{H}{d}$ or by increasing the flow rate. However, with high flow rates the mechanism of mass transfer for adsorption can shift from controlled by dispersion to diffusion, which may hinder the bed adsorption performance depending on adsorbent properties, hence emphasizing the importance of adsorbent selection (Thömmes et al., 1995a, 1995b). The hydrodynamic properties are further influenced by increased viscosity of the feedstock and presence of cells, discussed more in the next section.

Further parameters that can be obtained from the RTD data, applied generally to describe column efficiency for packed bed chromatography, include number of theoretical plates, *N*, and height equivalent of theoretical plate (HETP) defined as

$$N = 5.54\left(\frac{t_r}{W_{1/2}}\right)^2 \tag{11}$$

$$HETP = \frac{H}{N} \tag{12}$$

where $t_r$ is the retention time corresponding to time at maximum peak height, and $W_{1/2}$ is the peak width at half peak height.

Although parameters for expanded bed are usually determined uniform throughout the column height, in-bed monitoring studies have showed that within EBA column $\varepsilon$ and $D_{ax}$ vary depending on the axial height (Bruce and Chase, 2001; Lin et al., 2015; Willoughby et al., 2000). As a result of adsorbent classification, axial particle size decreases linearly by increase of axial height leading to increased axial voidage. Bruce and Chase (2001) reported that while the overall void fraction in an expanded bed with expansion rate of 2 was 0.70, the voidage in the top section of the column was 0.85 compared to 0.62 for the bottom section of the column determined from RTD tracer experiments. With a similar approach Lin et al. (2015) measured the local values for $N$ and HETP which increased and decreased, respectively, with increase of axial height under all test conditions. In general, a decrease in axial dispersion was observed with increase of axial height. However, after reaching a minimum value at a relative bed height of 0.6–0.8, the axial dispersion was reported to increase at the top part of the column due to high voidage causing deviation from plug flow (Fig. 6). As expected, due to larger mean particle size and increased axial dispersion at the bottom part of the column, significantly lower dynamic binding capacity was observed compared to top part of the bed which reached more than twice the capacity of the bottom section (Bruce and Chase, 2001). These differences along the column height become particularly important when attempting to model and predict the performance of EBA, unlike in packed beds, where hydrodynamic and adsorption parameters are not expected to show axial variation (Li et al., 2004).

Arpanaei et al. (2008) studied the differences of rotating (RFD) and localized stirring (LS) fluid distribution systems on hydrodynamic properties of EBA columns with diameters of 30, 60 and 150 cm. No significant difference was observed regarding column efficiency and degree of mixing when columns with 30 and 60 cm diameter were used, but with larger scale equipment the RFD outperformed the LS system, which suffered from reduced column efficiency and increased mixing described by Peclet number ($Pe$) that is similar to $Bo$, summarized in Fig. 7. Additionally, large EBA

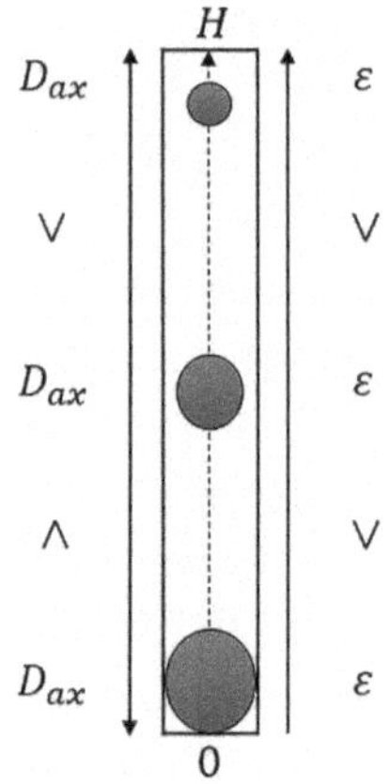


**Fig. 6** Axial variations for hydrodynamic properties in expanded bed column.

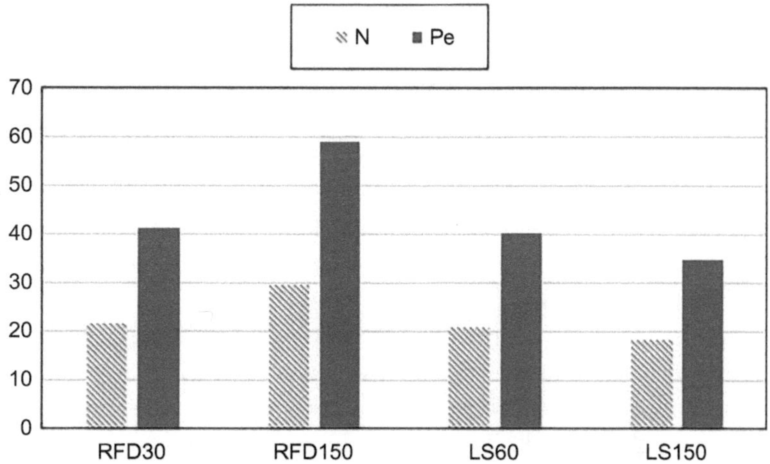


**Fig. 7** Comparison of hydrodynamic properties of EBA columns adapted with rotating fluid distributor (RFD) and local stirring (LS) fluid distribution system for column diameters of 30, 60 and 150 cm. *Data acquired from Arpanaei A, Heebøll-Nielsen A, Hubbuch JJ, Thomas, ORT, Hobley TJ: Critical evaluation and comparison of fluid distribution systems for industrial scale expanded bed adsorption chromatography columns.* J Chromatogr A, *1198–1199:131–139, 2008. doi:10.1016/j.chroma.2008.05.044.*

columns adapted with LS system suffered from dead zones and channeling under the distributor and between the baffles. Therefore, making rotating fluid distributors more suitable for designing large scale columns for EBA.

Further understanding of the hydrodynamic qualities of the column can be acquired by applying computational fluid dynamics (CFD). At an early stage of the process design CFD can be used for optimization of operating conditions to reduce the time and effort required for scale-up procedure (Koppejan et al., 2018).

## 3. Biomass-adsorbent interactions

Application of unclarified feedstock requires additional considerations for development of a downstream processing routine based on liquid-solid fluidized bed technology due to biomass-adsorbent interactions that are a major issue hindering robustness and efficiency of adsorption by changing hydrodynamic properties of the bed and decreasing binding capacity (Hubbuch et al., n.d.; Anspach et al., 1999; D'Souza et al., 2017). Biomass-adsorbent interactions may increase particle radius and lower density of the biomass covered particle, resulting in changed fluidization behavior of adsorbent particles, and lowered classification within the bed. Additionally, agglomerate formation can lead to channeling, and in worst case in collapse of the bed (Fernández-Lahore et al., 1999). Fouling of the adsorbent will decrease available binding sites for the target protein, hence hindering the adsorption capacity. However, severity of fouling, and therefore reduced capacity will depend on the nature of applied ligand. This was reported by Fernández-Lahore et al. (2000) and summarized in Fig. 8, showing that anion-exchangers are more prone to interact with negatively charged yeast cells compared to cation-exchangers.

In order to study the influence of biomass-adsorbent interactions for bed hydrodynamics, fluorescent tracers have been applied to overcome high background noise detected with spectrophotometer in the presence of biomass containing feedstock. To assess bed stability with clarified feedstock, the RTD data is commonly fitted to axially dispersed plug flow and tanks in series models. However, these models assume a homogenous distribution

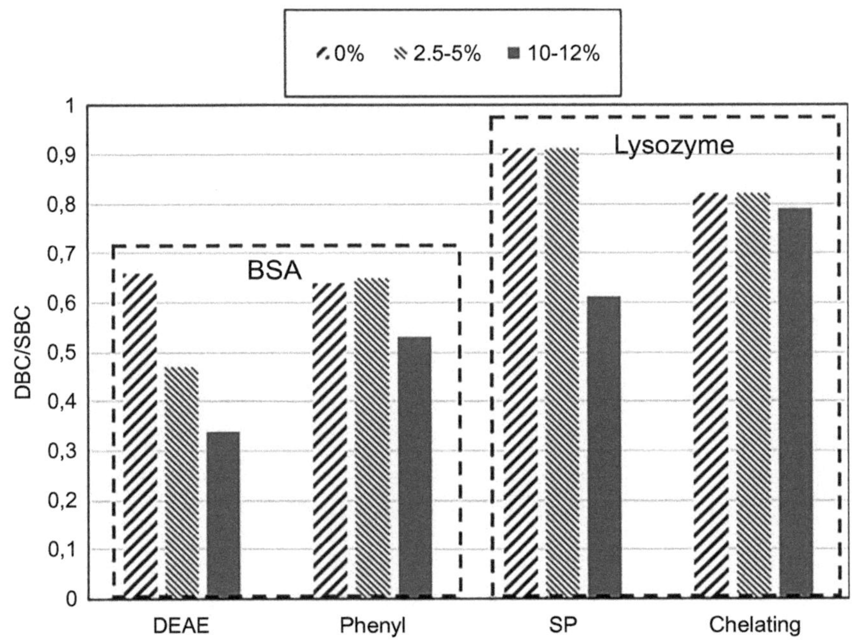


**Fig. 8** Ratios of dynamic (DBC) and static (SBC) binding capacity for adsorption of bovine serum albumin (BSA) onto Streamline DEAE and Phenyl, and adsorption of lysozyme onto Streamline SP and Chelating under varying percentage of yeast cell suspension. *Data acquired from Fernández-Lahore HM, Geilenkirchen S, Boldt K, Nagel A, Kula M, Thömmes J: The influence of cell adsorbent interactions on protein adsorption in expanded beds.* J Chromatogr A *873(2):195–208, 2000. doi:10.1016/S0021-9673(99)01308-4.*

of fluid throughout the system which is not valid for EBA due to formation of channeling, stagnant zones and possible adsorbent aggregation leading to a tailed pulse response curve. Therefore, Fernández-Lahore et al. (2000) analyzed the RTD data using axially dispersed plug-flow exchanging mass with stagnant zones (PDE) model provided by Villermaux and Van Swaaij (1969) in order to divide the bed into a perfectly classified and stable dynamic zone, and into a stagnant zone where fluidization properties deviate from ideal plug-flow. The PDE model characterizes the bed according to a fraction of stable expanded bed, $\phi$, a mass transfer term between both zones, $N$, and axial mixing in the stable zone using $Pe$ (Fig. 9) (Fernández-Lahore et al., 1999).

Increased fouling of weakly anionic Streamline DEAE was reported to lower the value of $\phi$ from 1 to 0.4 in comparison to 0.7 for strongly cationic Streamline SP as well as for Streamline Phenyl. With cation-exchangers $Pe$ numbers above 60 were obtained under all conditions, unlike with the anion-exchanger for which $Pe$ dropped down to 20 demonstrating how significantly the biomass-adsorbent interactions can influence the bed stability. (Fernández-Lahore et al., 2000).

## 3.1 Methods for the evaluation of adsorbent fouling

Finite bath experiments are performed to evaluate the degree of cell attachment onto stationary phase under static conditions by measuring the initial optical density of cell suspension with a UV detector at 600 nm and repeating the measurement after prolonged contact time with equilibrated stationary phase (Fernández-Lahore et al., 2000). The ratio between final, $OD_f$, and initial, $OD_i$, values for optical density are expressed as cell partition index (CPI) (Eq. 14) with a value of 1 corresponding to no cell attachment.

$$CPI = \frac{OD_f}{OD_i} \tag{13}$$

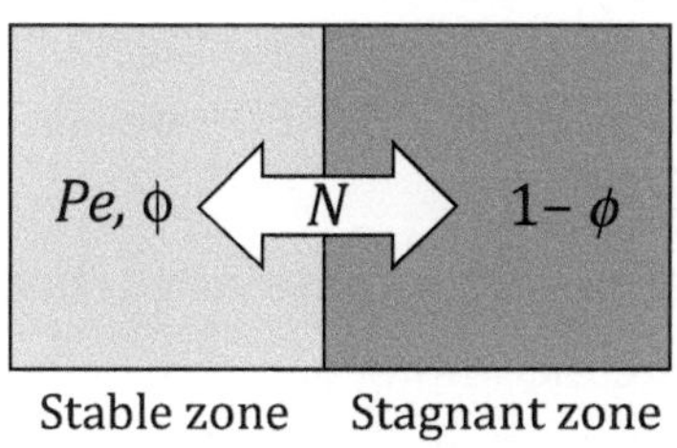


**Fig. 9** Schematic representation of the PDE model.

Similarly, the effect that cell attachment has on protein adsorption can be evaluated by adding moderate amount of cell suspension into a protein solution and measuring the initial absorbance at 280 nm and final absorbance after sufficient contact time with equilibrated adsorbent (Vennapusa and Fernandez-Lahore, 2010). The results are expressed according to Eq. 15 as an affinity number with a value of 0 corresponding to no protein adsorption taking place in the presence of cells.

$$\textit{Affinity number} = 1 - \frac{C_f}{C_i} \tag{14}$$

Biomass pulse technique is carried out under operational conditions by injecting a pulse of cell suspension into a fluidized bed and analyzing the UV response before and after the column. The degree of biomass-adsorbent interaction occurring is presented as the ratio between area of observed absorbance peak before and after the column (Feuser et al., 1999) Attachment efficiency, $\alpha$, is another parameter for evaluation of biomass-adsorbent interaction in the column, defined as ratio between experimentally determined deposition rate coefficient, $k_d$, and deposition rate coefficient under favorable electrostatic conditions, $k_{d,fav}$, determined by Redman et al. (2004) using a column packed with quartz grains that had been surface-modified with aminosilane to achieve non-repulsive behavior.

$$\alpha = \frac{k_d}{k_{d,fav}} \tag{15}$$

$$k_d = -\frac{U}{fL}\ln\left(\frac{C}{C_0}\right) \tag{16}$$

where $U$ is the superficial flow velocity, $f$, packed bed porosity, $L$ is the length of the packed bed, and $\frac{C}{C_0}$ is normalized breakthrough concentration. A methodological approach was presented by Lin et al. (2001) to minimize biomass-adsorbent interactions by applying the finite bath adsorption, biomass pulse response method, and RTD analysis. The combination of these methods reduced the development time significantly compared to the traditional "trial and error" method for EBA design.

## 3.2 Surface energetics of biomass-adsorbent interactions

The physical state of both the adsorbent and the solution environment have an effect on protein–surface as well as on biomass-surface interactions. In addition to hydrophobic interactions between the surface and colloidal particle, surface energy, charge and roughness are important factors influencing the interaction. (Hlady et al., 1999) The total interaction energy between a protein or biomass particle and a solid surface can be expressed according to the classical Derjaguin, Landau, Verwey, Overbeek (DLVO) theory which accounts for long-range electrodynamic Lifshitz–van der Waals (LW) and electrostatic interactions (EL). In the extended theory (XDLVO) short-range acid-base (AB) interactions, which accounts for the "hydrophobic attractive" as well as "hydrophilic repulsive" forces between colloidal particles, are also considered. The total interaction energy is expressed as the sum of all these interactions according to Eq. (17):

$$U_{mwc}^{XDLVO} = U_{mwc}^{LW} + U_{mwc}^{EL} + U_{mwc}^{AB} \tag{17}$$

Electrostatic interactions are the dominating force between adsorbent and biomass, and quantified using zeta-potential which is influenced by ionic conditions, pH, counterion concentration and its valence (Lin et al., 2003). In more detail the zeta-potential is defined as a potential difference between surrounding mineral-water interface and an external surface of a liquid layer of oppositely charged ions deposited onto a charged particle as illustrated in Fig. 10 (Branko et al., 1992). One of the most frequently applied electrokinetic techniques for obtaining zeta-potential values is

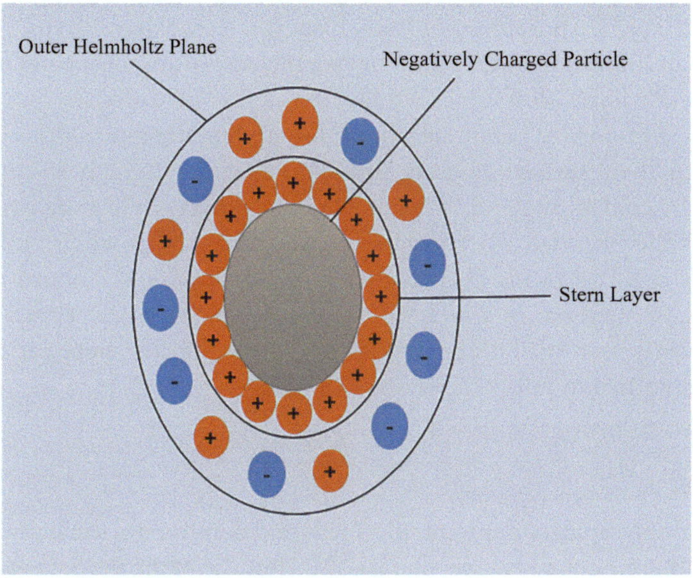


**Fig. 10** Gouy-Chapman-Stern model.

streaming potential measurement (Zembala, 2004). Streaming potential is the electrical potential difference across a stationary capillary or a porous plug, generated by displacement of the double layer ions in an electrolyte solution by applying a pressure gradient. Zeta-potential can be calculated employing streaming potential according to Eq. (18):

$$\zeta = \frac{dU_{str}}{d\Delta \mathrm{p}} \times \frac{\eta}{\varepsilon_0 \varepsilon} \kappa \tag{18}$$

where $U_{str}$ is the streaming potential, $\Delta$p is the pressure drop, $\eta$ is the viscosity and $\varepsilon_0\varepsilon$ is the dielectric coefficient of the electrolyte solution, and $\kappa$ is the electrical conductivity. Zeta potential is affected by the way the flow is damped in the vicinity of a solid surface and by geometrical morphology of the solid/liquid interface and therefore, for non-ideal interfaces the obtained value of zeta-potential has only relative meaning by giving some perception for the sign and magnitude of the part of the double-layer charge that controls the interaction between particles (Delgado et al., 2007; Zembala, 2004). The liquid layer is referred as Debye layer or electrical double layer (EDL). According to the Gouy-Chapman-Stern model the EDL is comprised of a Stern layer of adsorbed ions, and a diffuse layer, where the ions are arranged under the influence of electrical forces and thermal movements. The outer edge of the Stern layer is called the outer Helmholtz plane (OHP) (Kirby and Hasselbrink, 2004). Factors affecting the electric state of the Stern layer are properties of the solvent (dielectric permittivity), the surface group ionization degree and/or specific adsorption of species from the solution (Zembala, 2004).

Second important parameter for understanding the interactions of materials with their surroundings is surface wettability, which is commonly defined by contact angle of a liquid on a solid surface, indicating hydrophobicity of the material. To characterize wettability of powders and porous materials capillary rise is normally used, especially the Washburn capillary rise (WCR) method, in which the contact angle can be expressed in term of a squared mass of the penetrating liquid, *m*, and the penetrating time, *t*, according to Eq. (19):

$$\frac{m^2}{t} = \frac{c\rho^2 \sigma \cos\theta}{\eta} \tag{19}$$

where $c$ is the capillary constant, $\rho$ is the liquid density, $\sigma$ is the liquid surface tension, $\theta$ is the contact angle, and $\eta$ is the viscosity of the fluid. In the WCR method, the powder or porous material of interest is packed in a very narrow

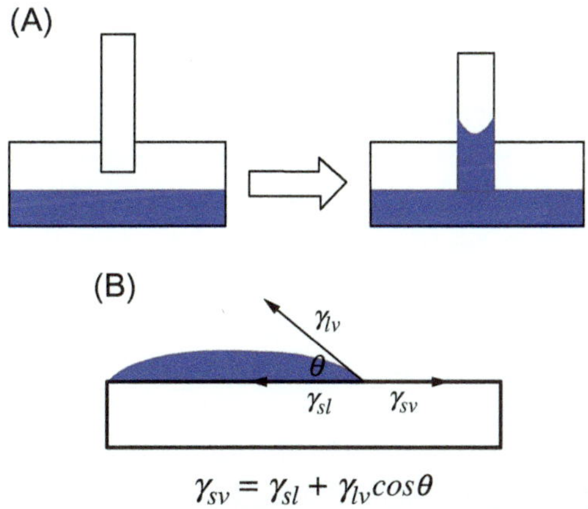


**Fig. 11** Measurement of contact angle with (A) capillary rise and (B) sessile drop method. *Adapted from Lazghab M, Saleh K, Pezron I, Guigon P, Komunjer L: Wettability assessment of finely divided solids.* Powder Technol, *157(1):79–91, 2005. doi:10.1016/j.powtec.2005.05.014.*

tube with a permeable bottom, which is immersed in a wetting liquid in order to determine the mass versus time data (Fig. 11A). Concerns regarding the WCR method are packing of the material and finding a suitable complete wetting liquid (cos $\theta = 0$) used for determining the capillary constant (Kirdponpattara et al., 2013). Additionally, Alghunaim and Newby reported on the hydrophobicity of the tubes having an effect on measured contact angles (Alghunaim and Zhang Newby, 2016). The contact angle for microbial cells is determined by applying sessile drop technique using the goniometer method (Sharma and Hanumantha Rao, 2002). In the method, a droplet is deposited by a syringe which is positioned above the sample surface, and a high resolution camera captures the image from the profile or side view (Fig. 11B).

Surface energy is a good predictor of biomass deposition onto surfaces and can be used as a diagnostic tool for evaluation of degree of fouling occurring with specific feedstock-adsorbent combinations, hence reducing the experimental efforts during EBA optimization (Li and Logan, 2004; Tari et al., 2008). Therefore, operational conditions can be adjusted to reduce adsorbent fouling (Vennapusa et al., 2008, 2009). Framework termed Interaction Energy Predictor (IntEP) was developed by D'Souza et al. to determine the most suitable mobile phase maximizing repulsion between biomass and adsorbent by employing the XDLVO theory to identify ideal pH and ionic strength conditions (D'Souza et al., 2017).

## 3.3 Additives to minimize biomass-adsorbent interactions

Various additives have been studied as a strategy to reduce the non-specific interactions of adsorbent with biomass either by adding directly to the feed stream or by coating the adsorbent to create a shielding layer. In comparison to hydrophobic and steric interactions, electrostatic forces are more significant during biomass-adsorbent interactions, and therefore non-ionic surfactants are able to function as an antifouling agent by increasing the electrostatic repulsion trough expansion of the electric double layer. (Brown and Jaffé, 2001; Galaev et al., 1994) The influence of various additives on cell deposition onto chromatographic support materials was reported by Vennapusa and Fernandez-Lahore (2010) who found polyvinyl pyrrolidone to have the most significant effect on adsorbent fouling by achieving approximately three fold reduction in cell attachment for Streamline DEAE in comparison to conditions without any additives (Fig. 12). The results were additionally confirmed with XDLVO calculations that had a good correlation with the experiments.

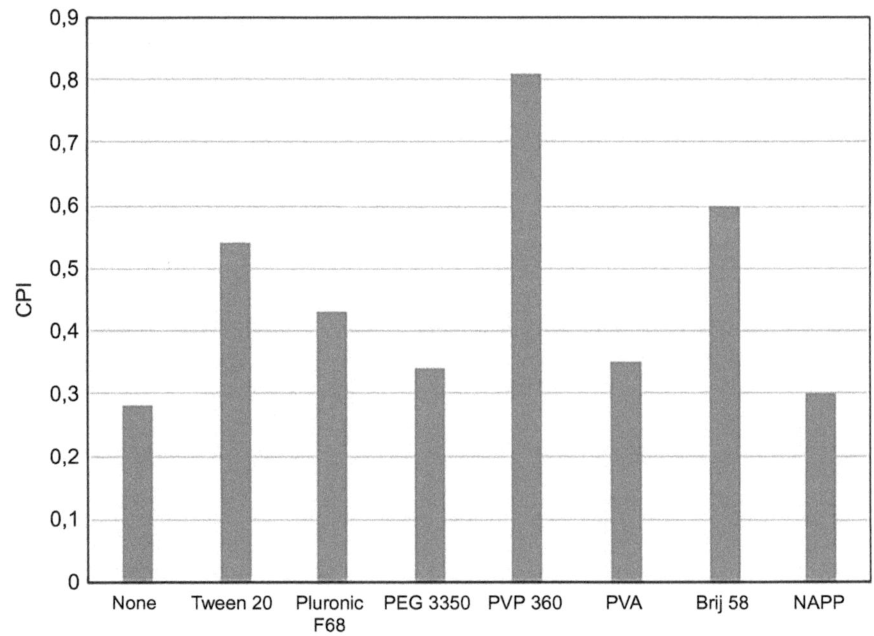


**Fig. 12** Deposition of yeast cells onto Streamline DEAE in the presence of various additives expressed with cell partition index. *Data acquired from Vennapusa RR, Fernandez-Lahore M: Effect of chemical additives on biomass deposition onto beaded adsorbents.* J Biosci Bioeng *110(5):564–571, 2010. doi:10.1016/j.jbiosc.2010.06.006.*

Hydrophilic polymers, such as poly(acrylic acid) (PAA), can be physically absorbed on the surface of the chromatographic support material to provide antifouling properties, and the physical characteristics of the coating, such as pore size and depth of polymer layer, can be modified according to the application (Dainiak et al., 2002; Jahanshahi et al., 2008). Dainiak et al. (2002, 2008) reported on light coating of PAA on adsorbent resulting in steep decline of biomass adsorption and in slight increase in static binding capacity when compared to the native adsorbent. However, a dense PAA coating prevented binding of protein onto the matrix. Bed expansion and hydrodynamic experiments conducted by Jahanshahi et al. (2008) demonstrated that polymer coated adsorbents can operate in similar conditions as native adsorbents. Additionally, employment of coated adsorbents resulted in lack of agglomerates leading to improved bed stability. Improved adsorption performance was also reported for expanded beds operated with PVP coated Streamline DEAE (Boeris et al., 2012; Vennapusa and Fernandez-Lahore, 2010).

## 4. Continuous downstream processing with solid-liquid fluidized bed technology

The switch from batch to continuous chromatography has been predominantly carried out by counter-current multicolumn chromatography systems such as simulated moving bed (SMB) chromatography (Angarita et al., 2015; Mueller et al., 2021; Nestola et al., 2015), and periodic counter current (PCC) chromatography (Godawat et al., 2012; Gomis-Fons et al., 2020). SMB chromatography is operated with two or more columns through which the fluid phase is flowing continuously and simultaneously the solid phase flow is simulated by periodically shifting the columns opposite to the fluid phase, improving the utilization of the stationary phase by achieving loadings much closer to the static binding capacity of the resin in comparison to batch chromatography, and reducing required column volume (Nestola et al., 2015). Similar to SMB, PCC system operates in a cyclic fashion by employing a column switching strategy which leads to continuous processing of the feed stream, while product elution from each column is discrete and periodic. PCC system is operated by overloading the first column and capturing the breakthrough on a second column leading to increased resin utilization in comparison to batch chromatography. The binding capacity of the resin determines the length of the load step, and therefore, the size and number of columns required for a given process are dependent of it. Compared to continuous PCC and SMB systems, counter current tangential chromatography (CCTC) allows the loading and elution of a product in a truly continuous and steady state fashion. All of the chromatographic steps are performed simultaneously and at steady state by flowing the resin slurry through a cascade of static mixers and hollow fiber membranes which retain the large resin particles while allowing dissolved species such as proteins to flow through. Additionally, the need for cleaning and cleaning validation can be eliminated with CCTC which employs a single-use flow path (Dutta et al., 2016). Multicolumn counter current solvent gradient purification (MCSGP) is a counter-current multicolumn technique specifically designed to be used for polishing step where many product-related impurities are present (De Luca et al., 2020). Operational principle of MCSGP is based on internal recycling of eluted fractions containing impurities between the columns which results in achieving increased yield while maintaining high purity. Therefore, the design of MCSGP process is based on batch chromatogram referred to as the "design chromatogram" which is obtained from single column batch operation (De Luca et al., 2020; Steinebach et al., 2017). The presented continuous chromatographic systems utilizing packed bed technology aren't suitable for unclarified feedstock, and therefore continuous systems utilizing liquid-solid fluidized bed technology could be applied for the initial capture step as a part of fully continuous DSP routine. Reported examples for continuous liquid-solid fluidized bed adsorption systems are discussed below.

## 4.1 Counter-current expanded bed system

The reported examples of EBA operating in a continuous mode were carried out using a system with an arrangement of counter current adsorption columns (Owen and Chase, 1997; Owen et al., 1997). In order to operate the adsorption process continuously, the expanded bed height is kept below the surface of the aqueous phase, which is removed at the top of the column. Adsorbent is constantly removed from the bottom part of the bed while adding adsorbent simultaneously at the top of the column, resulting in a downward flow of the adsorbent particles and achieving effective capture of the targeted protein. Similar to batch operation, feedstock is fed at the base of the column. The complete continuous protein purification system includes in total of four counter current columns, one for each stage of EBA process, arranged as shown in Fig. 13. The process streams are fed at the bottom of the column and become in contact with the falling

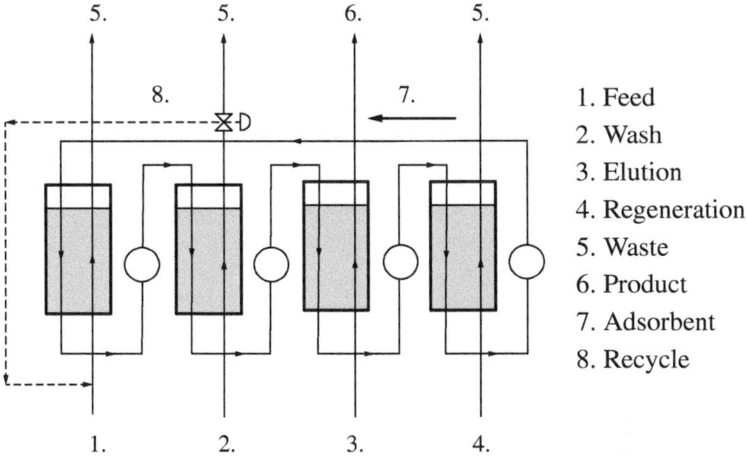


**Fig. 13** Schematic of continuous four-stage counter current EBA arrangement. *Adapted from Owen RO, McCreath GE, Chase HA: A new approach to continuous counter-current protein chromatography: direct purification of malate dehydrogenase from a Saccharomyces cerevisiae homogenate as a model system.* Biotechnol Bioeng *53(4):427–441, 1997. Retrieved from https://www.ncbi.nlm.nih.gov/pubmed/18634033.*

adsorbent particles. The aqueous phase leaves the column as a waste and adsorbent material is pumped to the next column. Before start-up of the continuous EBA process, each of the four columns were filled with the adsorbent either 20% or 30% of the total volume depending on the stage, and fluidized to reach a stable expanded bed height.

Successful application of the above-mentioned EBA arrangement is reported to achieve a yield of 90.5% with a purification factor of 19.4 for the purification of lysozyme from egg whites (Owen and Chase, 1997) and a yield of 78% with a purification factor around 10 for the purification of malate dehydrogenase from a *Saccharomyces cerevisiae* homogenate (Owen et al., 1997). A work aiming to develop a mathematical model for the counter current EBA column reported about impaired performance of the column as a result of adsorbent particle dispersion, which could be diminished by modifying the particle size distribution, resulting more closely to a plug-flow (Owen and Chase, 1999). Although the results were promising, the process was incapable of increasing the concentration of the targeted protein due to low ratio of the feed flowrate to eluant flowrate. Additionally, the necessary pumping and falling of adsorbent set mechanical constraints on adsorbent design, excluding support materials manufactured from agarose or other polysaccharides. Overall, the presented continuous

EBA arrangement is a promising premise for developing a continuous downstream process to address the needs of bioprocessing industry.

## 4.2 Liquid-solid circulating fluidized bed

Continuous protein capture from unclarified feedstock has been demonstrated using liquid-solid circulating fluidized bed (LSCFB) ion-exchange system by carrying out the protein adsorption in a downcomer and desorption in a riser as illustrated in Fig. 14 (Lan et al., 2000, 2002). The feed containing the product enters from the bottom part of the downcomer contacting down-ward moving adsorbent particles which after adsorption are transferred to the riser operated with a superficial fluid velocity greater than the terminal settling velocity of the adsorbent particles in order for them to reach the top part equipped with a liquid-solid separator. Main advantages of the LSCFB system include the integration of two columns into one system and process intensification achieved by high liquid-solid contact efficiency.

The downcomer has a height of 2.5 m with a diameter of 0.12 m, and the riser has a height of 3.0 m with a diameter of 0.038 m. The LSCFB system was successfully applied for recovery of bovine serum albumin (BSA) and whey protein isolate with a recovery around 90% in both cases and achieving

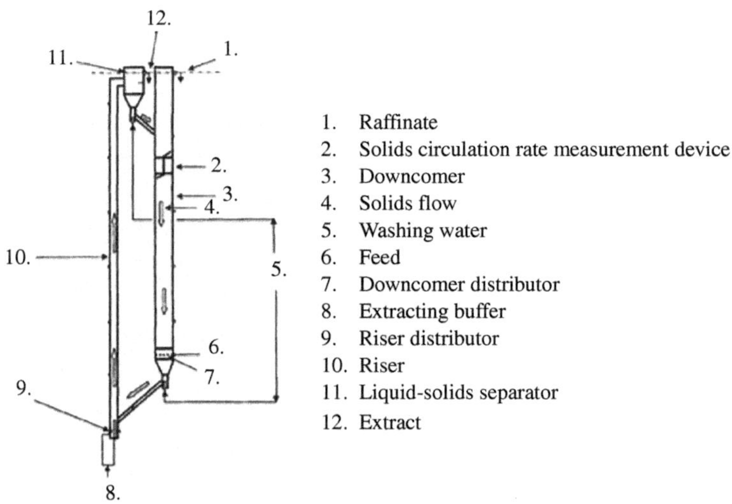


**Fig. 14** Schematic of liquid-solid circulating bed system. *Adapted from Lan Q, Zhu J, Bassi AS, Margaritis A, Zheng Y, Rowe GE: Continuous protein recovery using a liquid–solid circulating fluidized bed ion exchange system: modelling and experimental studies.* Can J Chem Eng *78(5):858–866, 2000. doi:10.1002/cjce.5450780502.*

productivity of 8.2 g/h of resin for latter. Despite successful recovery in the adsorption phase, the target protein concentration in effluent at outlet of riser was below the initial feedstock concentration, therefore suffering from same drawback as the counter-current EBA system (Lan et al., 2000, 2002).

## 5. Conclusions and future perspectives

Conventional downstream processing scheme suffers from complexity and long processing times which can be reduced through process intensification utilizing liquid-solid fluidized bed technology. Continuous manufacturing in the bioprocessing industry has been mostly focused on upstream processing where additionally increased titers have been achieved, shifting the bottleneck to downstream operations. Although liquid-solid fluidized bed technology hasn't gained much attention as a method for continuous processing, it offers advantages over packed bed technology and with further development could enable a way for more efficient bioprocessing.

## References

Abatari MN, Emami MRS, Jahanshahi M, Shahavi MH: Superporous pellicular κ-carrageenan–nickel composite beads: morphological, physical and hydrodynamics evaluation for expanded bed adsorption application, *Chem Eng Res Des* 125:291–305, 2017. https://doi.org/10.1016/j.cherd.2017.07.012.

Alghunaim A, Zhang Newby B: Influence of tube wettability on water contact angle of powders determined by capillary rise, *Colloids Surf A Physicochem Eng Asp* 492:79–87, 2016. https://doi.org/10.1016/j.colsurfa.2015.12.010.

Angarita M, Müller-Späth T, Baur D, Lievrouw R, Lissens G, Morbidelli M: Twin-column CaptureSMB: a novel cyclic process for protein A affinity chromatography, *J Chromatogr A* 1389:85, 2015. https://doi.org/10.1016/j.chroma.2015.02.046.

Anspach FB, Curbelo D, Hartmann R, Garke G, Deckwer W: *Expanded-bed chromatography in primary protein purification*, Netherlands, 1999, Elsevier B.V. https://doi.org/10.1016/S0021-9673(99)01119-X.

Arpanaei A, Heebøll-Nielsen A, Hubbuch JJ, Thomas ORT, Hobley TJ: Critical evaluation and comparison of fluid distribution systems for industrial scale expanded bed adsorption chromatography columns, *J Chromatogr A* 1198-1199:131–139, 2008. https://doi.org/10.1016/j.chroma.2008.05.044.

Asgari S, Jahanshahi M, Rahimpour A: Cost-effective nanoporous Agar–Agar polymer/nickel powder composite particle for effective bio-products adsorption by expanded bed chromatography, *J Chromatogr A* 1361:191–202, 2014. https://doi.org/10.1016/j.chroma.2014.08.016.

Asghari F, Jahanshahi M, Ghoreyshi AA: Preparation and characterization of agarose–nickel nanoporous composite particles customized for liquid expanded bed adsorption, *J Chromatogr A* 1242:35–42, 2012. https://doi.org/10.1016/j.chroma.2012.04.019.

Bermejo R, Ruiz E, Acien FG: Recovery of B-phycoerythrin using expanded bed adsorption chromatography: scale-up of the process, *Enzym Microb Technol* 40(4):927–933, 2007. https://doi.org/10.1016/j.enzmictec.2006.07.027.

Boeris V, Balce I, Vennapusa RR, Rodríguez MA, Picó G, Lahore MF: Production, recovery and purification of a recombinant β-galactosidase by expanded bed anion exchange adsorption, *J Chromatogr B* 900:32–37, 2012. https://doi.org/10.1016/j.jchromb.2012.05.024.

Branko S, Krasic D, Filipović S: *Measurement and application of zeta-potential*, 1992, Rudarsko-geološko-naftni fakultet Sveučilišta u Zagrebu. Retrieved from https://hrcak.srce.hr/24757.

Brown DG, Jaffé PR: Effects of nonionic surfactants on bacterial transport through porous media, *Environ Sci Technol* 35(19):3877–3883, 2001. https://doi.org/10.1021/es010577w.

Bruce LJ, Chase HA: Hydrodynamics and adsorption behaviour within an expanded bed adsorption column studied using in-bed sampling, *Chem Eng Sci* 56(10):3149–3162, 2001. https://doi.org/10.1016/S0009-2509(00)00549-2.

Chang Y, Chang I: Method development for direct recovery of lysozyme from highly crude chicken egg white by stirred fluidized bed technique, *Biochem Eng J* 30(1):63–75, 2006. https://doi.org/10.1016/j.bej.2006.02.006.

Chang YK, Chase HA: Development of operating conditions for protein purification using expanded bed techniques: the effect of the degree of bed expansion on adsorption performance, *Biotechnol Bioeng* 49:512–526, 1996. https://doi.org/10.1002/(SICI)1097-0290(19960305)49:53.0.CO;2-M.

Chase HA: Purification of proteins by adsorption chromatography in expanded beds, *Trends Biotechnol* 12(8):296–303, 1994. https://doi.org/10.1016/0167-7799(94)90046-9.

Chase HA, Draeger NM: Affinity purification of proteins using expanded beds, *J Chromatogr A* 597(1):129–145, 1992a. https://doi.org/10.1016/0021-9673(92)80103-2.

Chase HA, Draeger NM: Expanded-bed adsorption of proteins using ion-exchangers, *Sep Sci Technol* 27(14):2021–2039, 1992b. https://doi.org/10.1080/01496399208019462.

Chen K, Lee S, Show P, Hong S, Chang Y: Direct recovery of malate dehydrogenase from highly turbid yeast cell homogenate using dye-ligand affinity chromatography in stirred fluidized bed, *J Chromatogr B* 1100-1101:65–75, 2018. https://doi.org/10.1016/j.jchromb.2018.09.039.

Chen K, Chou S, Chang Y: Rapid purification of lysozyme by mixed-mode adsorption chromatography in stirred fluidized bed, *Food Chem* 272:619–627, 2019. https://doi.org/10.1016/j.foodchem.2018.06.050.

Chetty AS, Burns MA: Continuous protein separations in a magnetically stabilized fluidized bed using nonmagnetic supports, *Biotechnol Bioeng* 38(9):963–971, 1991. https://doi.org/10.1002/bit.260380902.

da Silva Padilha G, Curvelo-Santana JC, Alegre RM, Tambourgi EB: Expanded bed adsorption of an alkaline lipase from pseudomona cepacia, *J Chromatogr B* 877(5):521–526, 2009. https://doi.org/10.1016/j.jchromb.2008.12.061.

Dainiak MB, Galaev IY, Mattiasson B: Direct capture of product from fermentation broth using a cell-repelling ion exchanger, *J Chromatogr A* 942(1):123–131, 2002. https://doi.org/10.1016/S0021-9673(01)01345-0.

Dainiak MB, Galaev IY, Mattiasson B: Polyelectrolyte-coated ion exchangers for cell-resistant expanded bed adsorption, *Biotechnol Prog* 18(4):815–820, 2008. https://doi.org/10.1021/bp0202923.

De Luca C, Felletti S, Lievore G, et al.: Modern trends in downstream processing of biotherapeutics through continuous chromatography: the potential of multicolumn countercurrent solvent gradient purification, *Trends Anal Chem* 132, 2020, 116051. Retrieved from https://www.sciencedirect.com/science/article/pii/S0165993620302806.

Delgado AV, González-Caballero F, Hunter RJ, Koopal LK, Lyklema J: Measurement and interpretation of electrokinetic phenomena, *J Colloid Interface Sci* 309(2):194–224, 2007. https://doi.org/10.1016/j.jcis.2006.12.075.

D'Souza RN, Kakarla PB, Yelemane V, Meyer R, den Boer P, Fernández-Lahore M: Controlling cell adhesion in antibody purification by expanded bed adsorption chromatography, *Sep Purif Technol* 183:270–278, 2017. https://doi.org/10.1016/j.seppur.2017.03.002.

Dutta AK, Tan J, Napadensky B, Zydney AL, Shinkazh O: Performance optimization of continuous countercurrent tangential chromatography for antibody capture, *Biotechnol Prog* 32(2):430–439, 2016. https://doi.org/10.1002/btpr.2250.

Elmar H, Arno B, Charles C: *Development of sustainable bioprocesses*, West Sussex, England, 2006, John Wiley & Sons Ltd.

Fernández-Lahore HM, Kleef R, Kula M, Thömmes J: The influence of complex biological feedstock on the fluidization and bed stability in expanded bed adsorption, *Biotechnol Bioeng* 64(4):484–496, 1999. https://doi.org/10.1002/(SICI)1097-0290(19990820)64:43.0.CO;2-Z.

Fernández-Lahore HM, Geilenkirchen S, Boldt K, Nagel A, Kula M, Thömmes J: The influence of cell adsorbent interactions on protein adsorption in expanded beds, *J Chromatogr A* 873(2):195–208, 2000. https://doi.org/10.1016/S0021-9673(99)01308-4.

Feuser J, Walter J, Kula M, Thömmes J: Cell/adsorbent interactions in expanded bed adsorption of proteins, *Bioseparation* 8(1–5):99–109, 1999. https://doi.org/10.1007/978-94-017-1519-5_10.

Frej A, Johansson H, Johansson S, Leijon P: Expanded bed adsorption at production scale: scale-up verification, process example and sanitization of column and adsorbent, *Bioprocess Eng* 16:57–63, 1997. https://doi.org/10.1007/S004490050288.

Galaev IY, Garg N, Mattiasson B: Interaction of cibacron blue with polymers: Implications for polymer-shielded dye-affinity chromatography of phosphofructokinase from baker's yeast, *J Chromatogr A* 684(1):45–54, 1994. https://doi.org/10.1016/S0021-9673(94)89131-1.

Godawat R, Brower K, Jain S, Konstantinov K, Riske F, Warikoo V: Periodic counter-current chromatography—design and operational considerations for integrated and continuous purification of proteins, *Biotechnol J* 7(12):1496–1508, 2012. https://doi.org/10.1002/biot.201200068.

Gomis-Fons J, Andersson N, Nilsson B: Optimization study on periodic counter-current chromatography integrated in a monoclonal antibody downstream process, *J Chromatogr A* 1621, 461055, 2020. https://doi.org/10.1016/j.chroma.2020.461055.

Harrison RG, Todd P, Rudge SR, Petrides DP: *Bioseparations science and engineering*, 2003, Oxford University Press.

Hjorth R: Expanded-bed adsorption in industrial bioprocessing: recent developments, *Trends Biotechnol* 15(6):230–235, 1997. https://doi.org/10.1016/S0167-7799(97)01045-7.

Hlady, V., Buijs, J., & Jennissen, H. P. (1999). Methods for studying protein adsorption. Methods in enzymology (pp. 402–429). United States: Elsevier Science & Technology. doi:https://doi.org/10.1016/S0076-6879(99)09028-X Retrieved from https://www.sciencedirect.com/science/article/pii/S007668799909028X.

Hubbuch JJ, Heebøll-Nielsen A, Hobley TJ, Thomas ORT: A new fluid distribution system for scale-flexible expanded bed adsorption, *Biotechnol Bioeng* 78(1):35–43, 2002. https://doi.org/10.1002/bit.10170.

Hubbuch J., Thömmes J., Kula MR. Biochemical engineering aspects of expanded bed adsorption. In U. Kragl (Ed.), Technology transfer in biotechnology. Advances in biochemical engineering, vol 92. (pp. 101–123) Springer, Berlin, Heidelberg Retrieved from https://link.springer.com/book/10.1007%2Fb14094.

Jahanshahi M, Pacek AW, Nienow AW, Lyddiatt A: Fabrication by three-phase emulsification of pellicular adsorbents customised for liquid fluidised bed adsorption of bioproducts, *J Chem Technol Biotechnol* 78(11):1111–1120, 2003. https://doi.org/10.1002/jctb.907.

Jahanshahi M, Partida-Martinez L, Hajizadeh S: Preparation and evaluation of polymer-coated adsorbents for the expanded bed recovery of protein products from particulate feedstocks, *J Chromatogr A* 1203(1):13–20, 2008. Retrieved from https://www.sciencedirect.com/science/article/pii/S0190962218314385.

Karau A, Benken C, Thömmes J, Kula M: The influence of particle size distribution and operating conditions on the adsorption performance in fluidized beds, *Biotechnol Bioeng* 55(1):54–64, 1997. https://doi.org/10.1002/(SICI)1097-0290(19970705)55:13.0.CO;2-W.

Kirby BJ, Hasselbrink EF: Zeta potential of microfluidic substrates: 1. Theory, experimental techniques, and effects on separations, *Electrophoresis* 25(2):187–202, 2004. https://doi.org/10.1002/elps.200305754.

Kirdponpattara S, Phisalaphong M, Newby BZ: Applicability of Washburn capillary rise for determining contact angles of powders/porous materials, *J Colloid Interface Sci* 397:169–176, 2013. https://doi.org/10.1016/j.jcis.2013.01.033.

Koppejan V, Ferreira G, Lin D, Ottens M: Mathematical modelling of expanded bed adsorption—a perspective on in silico process design, *J Chem Technol Biotechnol* 93(7):1815–1826, 2018. https://doi.org/10.1002/jctb.5595.

Lan Q, Zhu J, Bassi AS, Margaritis A, Zheng Y, Rowe GE: Continuous protein recovery using a liquid–solid circulating fluidized bed ion exchange system: modelling and experimental studies, *Can J Chem Eng* 78(5):858–866, 2000. https://doi.org/10.1002/cjce.5450780502.

Lan Q, Bassi A, Zhu J, Margaritis A: Continuous protein recovery from whey using liquid-solid circulating fluidized bed ion-exchange extraction, *Biotechnol Bioeng* 78(2):157–163, 2002. https://doi.org/10.1002/bit.10171.

Lei Y, Lin D, Yao S, Zhu Z: Preparation of an anion exchanger based on TiO2-densified cellulose beads for expanded bed adsorption, *React Funct Polym* 62(2):169–177, 2005. https://doi.org/10.1016/j.reactfunctpolym.2004.08.004.

Levenspiel O: Chemical reaction engineering, *Ind Eng Chem Res* 38(11):4140–4143, 1999. https://doi.org/10.1021/ie990488g.

Li B, Logan BE: Bacterial adhesion to glass and metal-oxide surfaces, *Colloids Surf B: Biointerfaces* 36(2):81–90, 2004. https://doi.org/10.1016/j.colsurfb.2004.05.006.

Li P, Xiu G, Rodrigues AE: A 3-zone model for protein adsorption kinetics in expanded beds, *Chem Eng Sci* 59(18):3837–3847, 2004. https://doi.org/10.1016/j.ces.2004.06.008.

Lin DQ, Fernandez-Lahore HM, Kula M, Thömmes J: Minimising biomass/adsorbent interactions in expanded bed adsorption processes: a methodological design approach, *Bioseparation* 10:7–19, 2001. https://doi.org/10.1023/A:1012091031567.

Lin D, Brixius PJ, Hubbuch JJ, Thömmes J, Kula M: Biomass/adsorbent electrostatic interactions in expanded bed adsorption: a zeta potential study, *Biotechnol Bioeng* 83(2):149–157, 2003. https://doi.org/10.1002/bit.10654.

Lin D, Miao Z, Yao S: Expansion and hydrodynamic properties of cellulose-stainless steel powder composite matrix for expanded bed adsorption, *J Chromatogr A* 1107(1):265–272, 2006. https://doi.org/10.1016/j.chroma.2005.11.049.

Lin D, Shi W, Tong H, et al.: Evaluation and characterization of axial distribution in expanded bed: II. Liquid mixing and local effective axial dispersion, *J Chromatogr A* 1393:65–72, 2015. https://doi.org/10.1016/j.chroma.2015.03.019.

Mohsenkhani S, Jahanshahi M, Rahimpour A: Cross-linked κ-carrageenan polymer/zinc nanoporous composite matrix for expanded bed application: fabrication and hydrodynamic characterization, *J Chromatogr A* 1467:1, 2015. https://doi.org/10.1016/j.chroma.2016.09.018.

Mueller I, Seidel-Morgenstern A, Hamel C: Simulated-moving-bed technology for purification of the prebiotics galacto-oligosaccharides, *Sep Purif Technol* 271, 118829, 2021. https://doi.org/10.1016/j.seppur.2021.118829.

Nestola P, Silva RJS, Peixoto C, Alves PM, Carrondo MJT, Mota JPB: Robust design of adenovirus purification by two-column, simulated moving-bed, size-exclusion chromatography, *J Biotechnol* 213:109–119, 2015. https://doi.org/10.1016/j.jbiotec.2015.01.030.

Owen RO, Chase HA: Direct purification of lysozyme using continuous counter-current expanded bed adsorption, *J Chromatogr A* 757(1):41–49, 1997. https://doi.org/10.1016/S0021-9673(96)00680-2.

Owen RO, Chase HA: Modeling of the continuous counter-current expanded bed adsorber for the purification of proteins, *Chem Eng Sci* 54(17):3765–3781, 1999. https://doi.org/10.1016/S0009-2509(98)00477-1.

Owen RO, McCreath GE, Chase HA: A new approach to continuous counter-current protein chromatography: direct purification of malate dehydrogenase from a Saccharomyces cerevisiae homogenate as a model system, *Biotechnol Bioeng* 53(4):427–441, 1997. Retrieved from https://www.ncbi.nlm.nih.gov/pubmed/18634033.

Pålsson E, Gustavsson P, Larsson P: Pellicular expanded bed matrix suitable for high flow rates, *J Chromatogr A* 878(1):17–25, 2000. https://doi.org/10.1016/S0021-9673(00)00223-5.

Pessoa A, Hartmann R, Vitolo M, Hustedt H: Recovery of extracellular inulinase by expanded bed adsorption, *J Biotechnol* 51(1):89–95, 1996. https://doi.org/10.1016/0168-1656(96)01573-8.

Redman JA, Walker SL, Elimelech M: Bacterial adhesion and transport in porous media: role of the secondary energy minimum, *Environ Sci Technol* 38(6):1777–1785, 2004. https://doi.org/10.1021/es034887l.

Rezvani A, Jahanshahi M, Najafpour GD: Characterization and evaluation of the novel agarose–nickel composite matrix for possible use in expanded bed adsorption of bio-products, *J Chromatogr A* 1331:61–68, 2014. https://doi.org/10.1016/j.chroma.2014.01.026.

Richardson JF, Zaki WN: Sedimentation and fluidisation 1. Institution of chemical engineers, *Trans Inst Chem Eng* 32(1):35–52, 1954.

Safarik I, Safarikova M: Magnetic techniques for the isolation and purification of proteins and peptides, *Biomagn Res Technol* 2(1):7, 2004. https://doi.org/10.1186/1477-044X-2-7.

Sharma PK, Hanumantha Rao K: Analysis of different approaches for evaluation of surface energy of microbial cells by contact angle goniometry, *Adv Colloid Interf Sci* 98(3):341–463, 2002. https://doi.org/10.1016/S0001-8686(02)00004-0.

Show PL, Ooi CW, Song CP, et al.: Purification of lysozyme from chicken egg white by high-density cation exchange adsorbents in stirred fluidized bed adsorption system, *Food Chem* 343, 128543, 2021. https://doi.org/10.1016/j.foodchem.2020.128543.

Shukla AA, Etzel MR, Gadam S: *Process scale bioseparations for the biopharmaceutical industry*, 2007, Taylor & Francis Group.

Silvino Dos Santos E, Guirardello R, Teixeira Franco T: Preparative chromatography of xylanase using expanded bed adsorption, *J Chromatogr A* 944(1):217–224, 2002. https://doi.org/10.1016/S0021-9673(01)01368-1.

Song CP, Ooi CW, Tey BT, Lu C, Liu B, Chang Y: Direct recovery of enhanced green fluorescent protein from unclarified escherichia coli homogenate using ion exchange chromatography in stirred fluidized bed, *Int J Biol Macromol* 164:4455–4465, 2020. https://doi.org/10.1016/j.ijbiomac.2020.09.051.

Steinebach F, Ulmer N, Decker L, Aumann L, Morbidelli M: Experimental design of a twin-column countercurrent gradient purification process, *J Chromatogr A* 1492:19–26, 2017. https://doi.org/10.1016/j.chroma.2017.02.049.

Tari C, Vennapusa R, Cabrera RB, Fernández-Lahore M: Colloid deposition experiments as a diagnostic tool for biomass attachment onto bioproduct adsorbent surfaces, *J Chem Technol Biotechnol* 83(2):183–191, 2008. https://doi.org/10.1002/jctb.1852.

Thömmes J, Halfar M, Lenz S, Kula M: Purification of monoclonal antibodies from whole hybridoma fermentation broth by fluidized bed adsorption, *Biotechnol Bioeng* 45(3):205–211, 1995a. https://doi.org/10.1002/bit.260450304.
Thömmes J, Weiher M, Karau A, Kula MR: Hydrodynamics and performance in fluidized bed adsorption, *Biotechnol Bioeng* 48(4):367–374, 1995b. https://doi.org/10.1002/bit.260480409.
Thömmes J, Bader A, Halfar M, Karau A, Kula M: Isolation of monoclonal antibodies from cell containing hybridoma broth using a protein A coated adsorbent in expanded beds, *J Chromatogr A* 752(1–2):111–122, 1996. https://doi.org/10.1016/S0021-9673(96)00504-3.
Tong X, Sun Y: Application of magnetic agarose support in liquid magnetically stabilized fluidized bed for protein adsorption, *Biotechnol Prog* 19(6):1721–1727, 2003. https://doi.org/10.1021/bp030028p.
Vennapusa RR, Fernandez-Lahore M: Effect of chemical additives on biomass deposition onto beaded adsorbents, *J Biosci Bioeng* 110(5):564–571, 2010. https://doi.org/10.1016/j.jbiosc.2010.06.006.
Vennapusa R, Hunegnaw SM, Cabrera RB, Fernández-Lahore M: Assessing adsorbent–biomass interactions during expanded bed adsorption onto ion exchangers utilizing surface energetics, *J Chromatogr A* 1181(1):9–20, 2008. https://doi.org/10.1016/j.chroma.2007.11.078.
Vennapusa RR, Tari C, Cabrera R, Fernandez-Lahore M: Surface energetics to assess biomass attachment onto hydrophobic interaction adsorbents in expanded beds, *Biochem Eng J* 43(1):16–26, 2009. https://doi.org/10.1016/j.bej.2008.08.004.
Villermaux J, Van Swaaij WPM: Modèle représentatif de la distribution des temps de séjour dans un réacteur semi-infini à dispersion axiale avec zones stagnantes. application à l'écoulement ruisselant dans des colonnes d'anneaux raschig, *Chem Eng Sci* 24(7):1097–1111, 1969. https://doi.org/10.1016/0009-2509(69)80081-3.
Willoughby NA, Hjorth R, Titchener-Hooker NJ: Experimental measurement of particle size distribution and voidage in an expanded bed adsorption system, *Biotechnol Bioeng* 69(6):648–653, 2000. AID-BIT9 > 3.0.CO;2-U.
Xia H, Lin D, Yao S: Chromatographic performance of macroporous cellulose–tungsten carbide composite beads as anion-exchanger for expanded bed adsorption at high fluid velocity, *J Chromatogr A* 1195(1):60–66, 2008. https://doi.org/10.1016/j.chroma.2008.04.080.
Zembala M: Electrokinetics of heterogeneous interfaces, *Adv Colloid Interf Sci* 112(1):59–92, 2004. https://doi.org/10.1016/j.cis.2004.08.001.
Zhou X, Sun Y, Liu Z: Superporous pellicular agarose–glass composite particle for protein adsorption, *Biochem Eng J* 34(2):99–106, 2007. https://doi.org/10.1016/j.bej.2006.09.018.
Zuwei J: Expanded bed adsorption—challenges and advances in column and process design, *Pharm Eng* 35:66–78, 2015.

CHAPTER FIVE

# Smart platform for development of small-scale integrated continuous downstream processes

**Niklas Andersson, Joaquín Gomis Fons, and Bernt Nilsson***
Department of Chemical Engineering, Lund University, Lund, Sweden
*Corresponding author: e-mail address: bernt.nilsson@chemeng.lth.se

## Contents



## Abstract

This chapter presents and discuss a platform for small-scale drug candidate production, process development and performance studies of integrated continuous downstream processes. The main idea of the platform methodology is to use common available equipment and reconfigure them for advanced downstream processing. Five different industrial case studies are discussed. The resulting processes are automated and controlled by the external supervisory controller, called Orbit. Orbit communicate with the local equipment control system, resulting in a minimum of adjustment in the laboratory infrastructure. Orbit is implemented in python, making it an open, flexible, and extendable control system. Orbit give support for integration of multiple chromatography columns, operate downstream processes on multiple parallel setups, integrated online analytics, use of advanced feedback control and batch-to-batch control. This functionality is presented in ten examples. The platform has successful been used in number of industrial case studies, particular in early drug and process development and for efficient small-scale drug candidate production.

*Advances in Chemical Engineering*, Volume 59
ISSN 0065-2377
https://doi.org/10.1016/bs.ache.2022.03.004

## 1. Introduction

The introduction of process intensification and continuous processing of biologics in the biopharmaceutical industry creates a need for new tools and methodologies for drug and process development (Farid, 2007; Kesik-Brodacka, 2018; Konstantinov and Cooney, 2015; Shukla et al., 2017; Shukla and Thömmes, 2010; Walther et al., 2015; Zydney, 2015). There is an ongoing discussion where to introduce integrated continuous operation, process intensification and advanced monitoring and control, in the process development chain. In principle there are two ways, as late as possible or as early as possible. The benefit of late introduction means that the traditional development chain can be left unchanged and final process is redesigned into an intensified and continuous version for commercial production. The drawback is the loss of time for reconfiguration and filing of a new process design. The alternative is to introduce these concepts already in early development and to base all process development and validation on integrated continuous process design. The drawback is the need to change the methodology in the process development chain, from early process designs for drug candidates, via pilot validations for clinical trials, to process design for commercial production.

To introduce advanced processing already in early drug development, the methodology and tools have to be adjusted for flexible small-scale studies and multiple drug candidate production. This results in the need of a platform that is open, flexible, extendable, scalable, and fully automated. The platform that is presented here is based on the following design criteria:

- exploit common available equipment and their local control software, here exemplified by different ÄKTA and Agilent systems, and use software communication for automation and control.
- add minor equipment, like scale, stirrer, heater, external detectors, and use serial communication.
- flexible and extendable automation using a supervisory control system that orbits the physical process configuration, and makes it easy to study and change different process configurations.
- open architecture for the design of advanced process control for performance and quality control.
- scalable process design and automation system from small-scale in early development to pilot-scale in process validation.

An important element in a control strategy is to have a supervisory control and data acquisition (SCADA) software in order to integrate the software and hardware of different units. The research software Orbit has been developed to be a general control software for sequential control, data acquisition and advanced real-time supervisory controller, for lab-scale process development. Orbit was originally created to control the chromatography systems ÄKTA™ to overcome the limitations of the ÄKTA control system UNICORN™. Unlike the latter control system, Orbit allows the simultaneous control of several systems and analytical equipment, the use of real-time control, and the implementation of complex automation strategies. Orbit, written in python language, communicates with UNICORN to send instructions at determined times and receive data from the system, based on the information provided by the user about the process.

The main idea is to use an open, flexible, and extendable computing environment that also have the capability to communicate in real-time with equipment. Orbit is based on python, which gives the user a large library of computational tools. There is a number of good alternatives, like MATLAB (Feidl et al., 2020), Java and Julia, that gives similar capabilities. The opposite idea is to base the platform on a well-established automation software, like DeltaV or similar software's. These software's gives the user a complete solution for process automation which is capable to scale from early development to commercial production. The drawback are the investment cost and the flexibility for reconfigurations (Fig. 1).

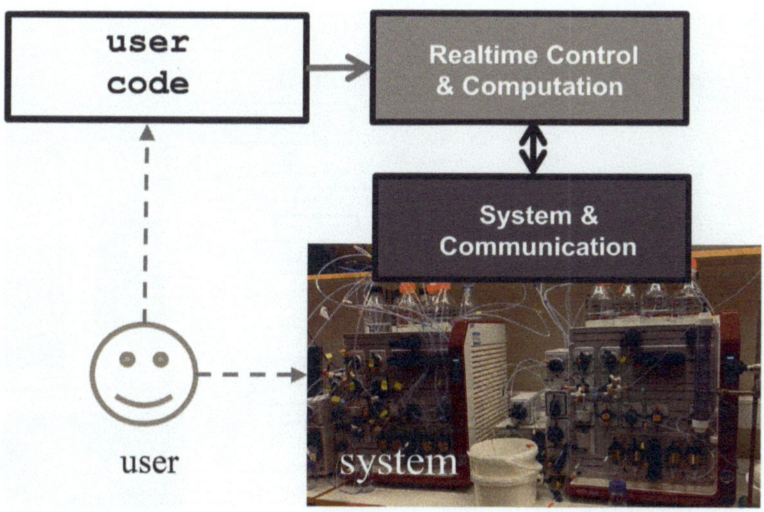


**Fig. 1** Overall principle behind the platform.

## 2. Orbit platform concept

The need for an open, flexible and extendable environment for the operation, automation and control of advanced downstream processes was the origin for the development of the research software Orbit (Andersson et al., 2017). The first applications were to use an ÄKTA system as the physical process and control Unicorn from the outside. This was done already back in 2015 in python 2, and with the latest version orbit in python 3 (2020). In Fig. 1 the user interacts with the physical system and writes user code to define configuration and the sequence of operations. The real-time controller then execute the user code and communicate with the physical system.

Orbit is a general controller that can control any equipment that offers a communication protocol that is supported in python. Instruments run by Unicorn can be controlled by OPC or a REST API. Orbit also supports serial communication (RS232), which is common among many instruments such as balances, heaters, sensors and stirrers. Agilent instruments offer control through an API called Instrument Communication Framework (ICF), and this is implemented as a communication extension, called Satellite, for the control of HPLC setups and advanced detectors. The list of equipment that has been controlled with orbit includes ÄKTA (pure, avant, pcc, explorer, purifier), Agilent 1260, KrosFlo, scales, stirrer, syringe pump, valves.

An overview of the orbit structure can be seen in Fig. 2, where the user writes code that is sent to the orbit kernel. This is the digital system

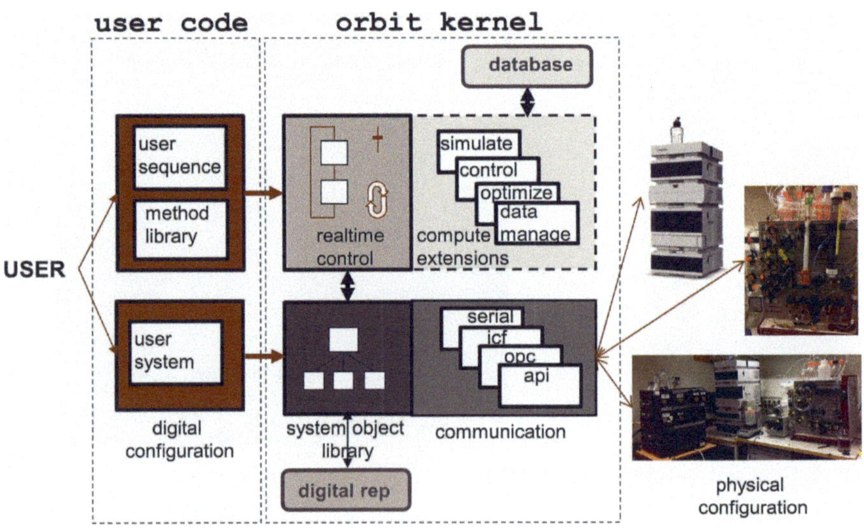


Fig. 2 Orbit software architecture.

configuration and the sequence of phases to be run in the process. The orbit kernel contains the realtime control part and the system object library part that communicates with the physical system.

In the realtime control, called orbit process, all logics and instructions are handled. The user defines the phases to be run either sequentially or in parallel. The phases include time or state-based events that are checked and when fired, the action is executed. The action can be simple instructions but can also be dynamic advanced functions. The kernel also handles all data collection, synchronization and monitoring. It is possible to add parallel loops for control or other tasks. The kernel can easily be extended with extensions such as simulation, optimization or database communication.

The orbit kernel contains the system representation with a unit library with methods for control of the physical system. The user sets up all the unit of the process in a system configuration where instances of all units are built. The user can connect everything with tubes to let orbit know the flow paths in the process. The units contain methods like get and set for control.

A process is designed as a sequence of phases with information on the commands to execute and when to trigger them. They can be triggered based on a specified time or for an event to occur specified as a logic. The phases can be arranged to run in parallel with possibility to add points of synchronization. In Fig. 3 an example is shown where a process is started in sequence and then split in parallel to set a gradient profile in one branch and the pooling strategy in the other. All phases are defined with events and actions defined and is assembled with lists and sent to the Orbit process.

## 3. Platform for integrated downstream process development

In early product and process development, it is desired to both test and verify process configurations and to perform small-scale production of a drug candidate for further candidate studies. In this situation it is convenient to use only one experimental setup that can handle an integrated downstream process, due to limited resource for many drug candidates. This means that a complete downstream process, with multiple purifications steps, is configured and operated in sequence. The basic idea is to run each purification step as it is supposed to be operated as stand-alone. The main difference is that the product pool is directed to the next purification step and loaded directly. After the pooling the first step is parked and the separation procedure starts the processing of the second step, which is in its turn is parked after pooling. This goes on to the last purification step when the product is pooled. After product pooling the columns can be regenerated and equilibrated one after

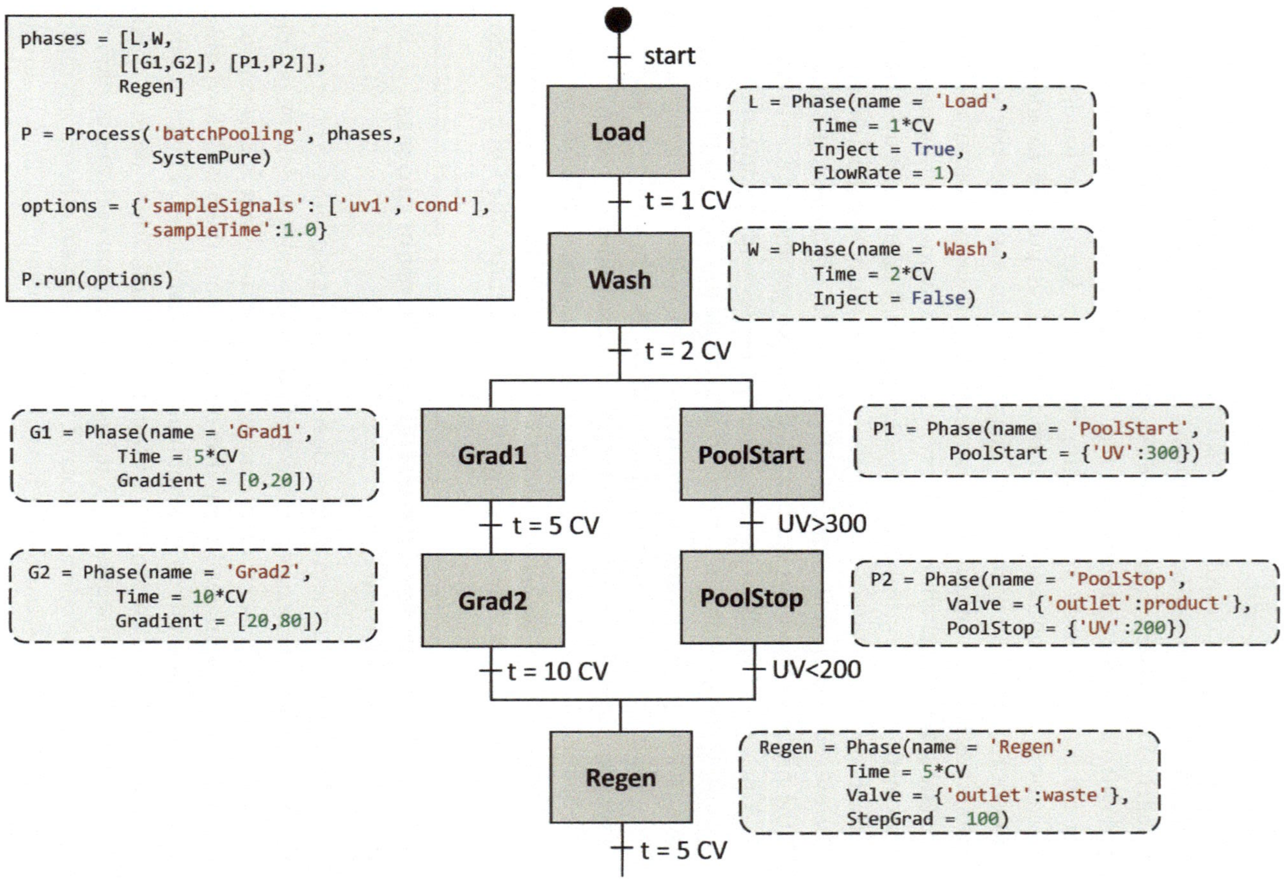


**Fig. 3** A simple process example in orbit with pooling and multigradient implemented in parallel.

the other. An alternative is of course to clean the columns after pooling and park the pool in the next column. Here the design is to minimize the hold-up time for the product in the downstream process and therefore all columns are parked after pooling. This was is presented in Andersson et al. (2017), Gomis-Fons et al. (2019), Löfgren et al. (2018).

The configuration of an integrated downstream process on one experimental setup is seen in Fig. 4. The configuration is implemented on one ÄKTA pure system, from Cytiva, but can also be configured in a similar way on other comparable liquid chromatography systems. The basic configuration is indicated by solid lines. The gradient pump, with it's A and B pumps, is connected, via the injection valve, InjV, for feed of sample to a versatile valve, VV1. This valve directs the flow to the column valve, CV, or to the loop valve, LV. Odd columns are connected to the loop valve and even to the column valve. After these two valves a second versatile valve, VV2, directs the flow to waste or to the train of detectors ending at the outlet valve, OV. This means that when a column is washed and eluted the buffers

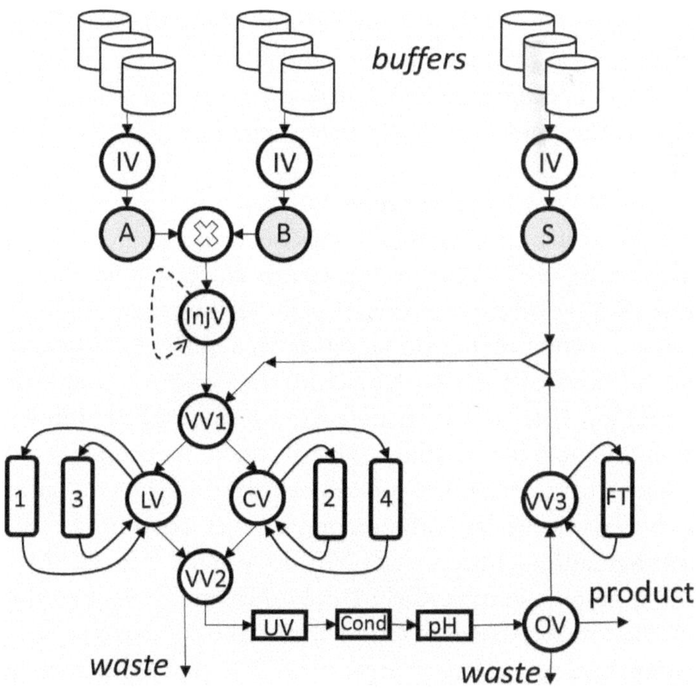


**Fig. 4** The configuration of integrated column sequence on one experimental setup with four column/loop positions, 1–4, and one flow-through position, FT.

are pump by the gradient pump through the first and second versatile valves, to the outlet valve for switching between waste, recycle or product. Product is the pool from the last column, while recycle is the intermediate pool from previous step to the next. If the eluting column is odd the pool is loaded on to an even column, therefore the ordering of columns on the loop and column valves. When the next column is eluted on the column valve, its pool will be directed to the next column in the sequence connected to the loop valve.

To make it possible to load a previous pool onto the next column it often needs to be conditioned. Here we have solved it by in-line dilution of the pool by using the sample pump, and this is done in the recycle flow path from the outlet valve to the first versatile valve. This general configuration can handle up to 10 bind-and-elute chromatography steps in a sequence, with on-line dilution as conditioning between the steps.

On the recycle flow path a third versatile value is added, making it possible to also integrate a flow-through step in the downstream processing. One limitation is that the configuration only has one conditioning possibility, meaning that the flow path can only be conditioned before or after the flow through step. In Fig. 4 it is conditioned after the flow through step. If conditioning is also needed of the pool from the step before, a buffer exchange column needs to be introduced as an extra column in the column sequence, and the pool from the buffer exchanger is loaded on the flow through step.

The integrated downstream process discussed above, and seen in Fig. 4, runs all separation steps in a sequence. This can be done once, just producing one pool, or multiple times processing a larger amount of feed. For this purpose, there are three different alternatives for feeding the process, illustrated in an extended version of the configuration seen in Fig. 5. The basic feeding is by using the injection valve with one injection loop or multiple times with a larger superloop. A second alternative is to use one of the pumps to load the first column. In Fig. 5 this is indicated by the use of the sample pump, feed2. For continuous feed, feed3, the process needs a minor reconfiguration. By adding two versatile valves and a second capture column, a twin capture column configuration is introduced on the loop valve. This makes it possible to load the capture column and elute the other one. Note that the loading time of the capture step needs to be larger than the complete processing time of the rest of the downstream process. Note also that experimental setup is limited to only four versatile valves, meaning that a twin capture column configuration cannot be configured together with a flow through step.

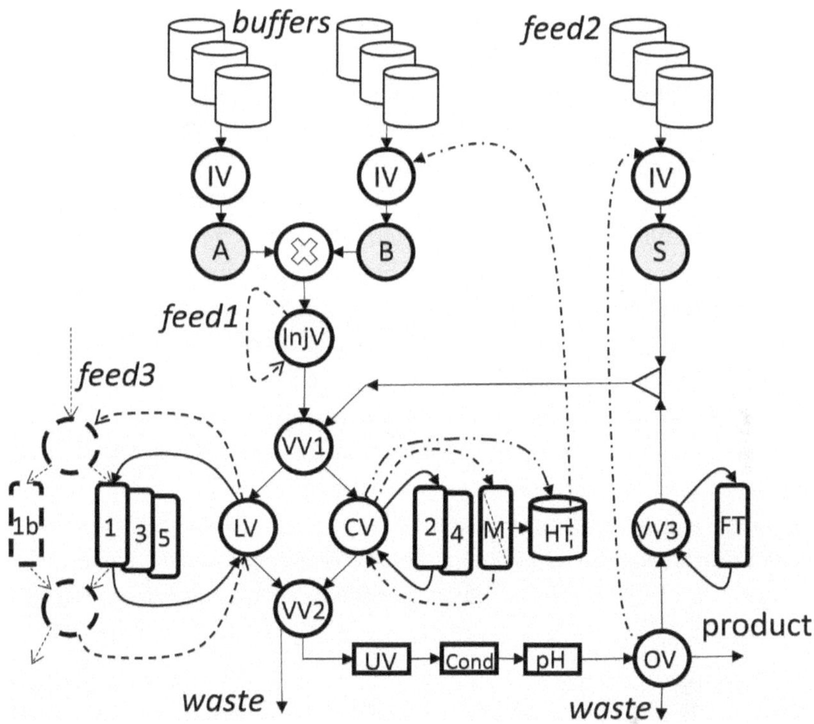


**Fig. 5** The general configuration of integrated downstream process. The configuration has five column positions, one flow-through position, three possible feed positions; position for UFDF step, which also can be used as batch reactor position.

In some situations, the product needs to be processed further in a formulation step, for instance ultrafiltration and diafiltration step, UFDF. The pool from the last separation step is directed to the hold-up tank, HT, for the UFDF-step, indicated by the dashed-dotted lines in Fig. 5. The pump B suck the hold-up tank liquid through the system to the column value in the membrane, M, and the retentate goes back to the hold-up tank. The permeate pass through the membrane caused by the sample pump, via the through versatile valve two and the outlet valve. The trans-membrane pressure can be measured by the build in column valve pressure sensor. This is how ultrafiltration can be performed. Diafiltration and buffer change is performed by the use of pump A for the addition of formulation buffer. Note that the membrane configuration presented here can be used as a conditioning step anywhere in a downstream process sequence and can be added to the discussion above about conditioning of the recycle flow.

The hold-up tank can also be used as a chemical reactor position. The pool from a chromatography step is pumped to the hold-up tank. The hold-up tank can be complemented by stirrer, scale and heater, controlled by Orbit using serial communication of external hardware. Reactants can be added by the system through the three pumps or additional external pumps, like syringe pumps. Number of different reactions can be performed in this way, like viral inactivation and reactions for protein modifications, tagging or cleavage. When the time for the reaction is out the content is pumped to further processing in the sequence.

**Example 1.** *Integration of five step downstream process*

*A therapeutic protein is purified in five step downstream process* (Gomis-Fons et al., 2019). *The first step is a mixed mode column with high specificity for the target protein, followed by three purification steps, two ion exchangers with an active membrane adsorption in between. The flow sheet is seen in Fig. 6 and the configuration on one experimental setup is seen in Fig. 5, with the mixed-mode and anion exchanger as odd columns 1 and 3, and the cation exchanger and the ultrafiltration as even steps 2 and UFDF. The membrane is positioned as a flow-through step at FT.*

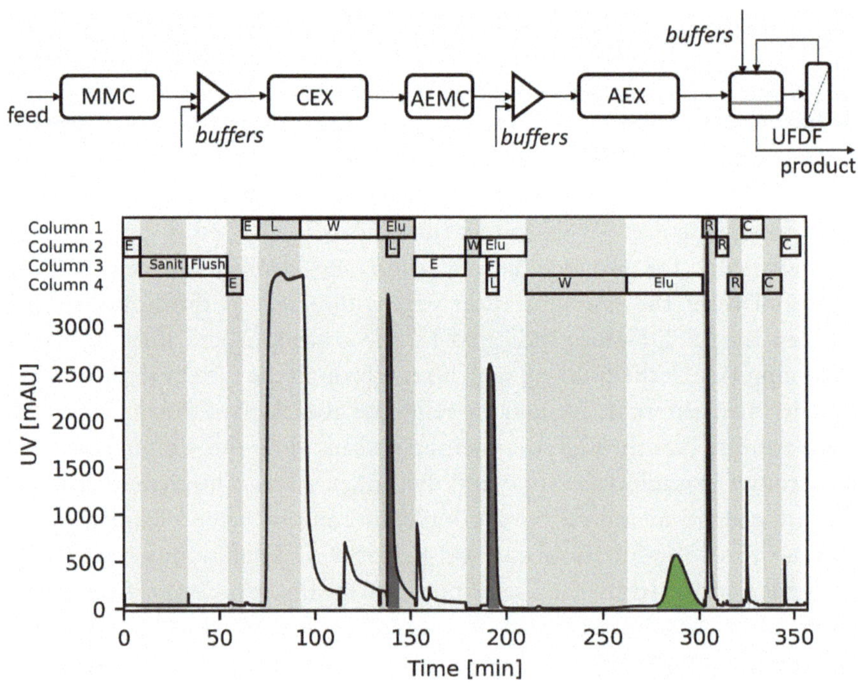


**Fig. 6** The downstream process in Example 1, (above) The principle process diagram, (below) The complete chromatogram for the four separation steps.

*The UV signal from the sequence of adsorption steps is seen in Fig. 6, where the individual pools from each separation steps are filled. In-line dilution is done between step one and two and between step three and four. Note that the membrane adsorber run in flow through mode so the target goes directly to the final ion exchanger, without passing the detectors Fig. 6.*

*Finally, the downstream process has a membrane process for buffer exchange and concentration. In this study the product pool first was concentrated, followed by sequential diafiltration, and ends with a second concentration. The configuration used in this work had limited flexibility forcing the diafiltration to operate sequential. Note that the UFDF configuration seen in Fig. 5 allow for continuous diafiltration. The membrane process configuration on the experimental setup as shown here need some extra attention. The transmembrane pressure can be measured using the pressure detector in the column valve but the retentate pressure needs to be measured by an external pressure detector. The trans-membrane pressure is controlled by a PI-controller in Orbit by the changing the flow rate. In relation to this there is a need for a pressure value on the retentate side and here this pressure valve has been a simple manual valve for manual control of the retentate pressure (Fig. 7).*

## 4. Small-scale continuous downstream processing

Chromatography that is based on packed bed columns operate batchwise and the feed and product stream are periodic. By connecting multiple columns the feed to the chromatography step can be continuous, but

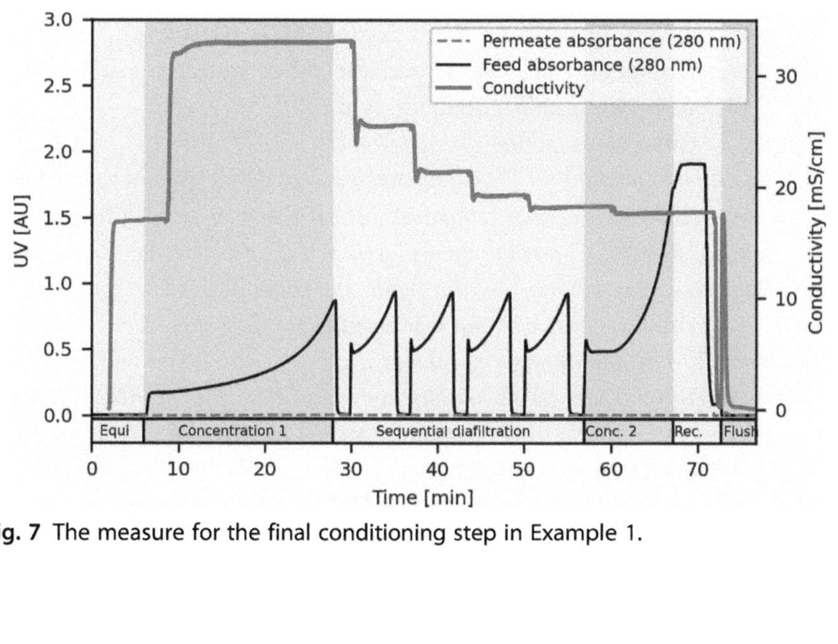


**Fig. 7** The measure for the final conditioning step in Example 1.

the product is still periodic. If it is important to have a continuous product flow the step needs to add a hold-up tank after the chromatography column. A straightforward way is to run a set of columns in parallel that results in continuous feed. Twin column capture, with loading times longer than the rest of the cycle, makes it possible to run continuously. This is used in an example below.

To increase the productivity further, introduction of more efficient capture steps is needed, like periodic counter current system, PCC, or capture simulated moving bed, capture SMB (Baur et al., 2016a, 2016b; Godawat et al., 2012; Riske and Ransohoff, 2017; Shi et al., 2021). These systems are more complicated and needs to be operated on one setup by its own. This makes it possible to run the downstream process in parallel. An implementation of a 3-column PCC configuration on one ÄKTA pure setup is seen in Fig. 9 (Gomis-Fons et al., 2020a). A similar configuration of capture SMB on one experimental setup is found in (Moreno-González et al., 2021). Other process intensification chromatography setups have been studied by this framework. Multi-column counter-current solvent gradient purification, MCSGP, and similar version as twin column recycling, TCR, has been configured and controlled by the Orbit software (Gomis-Fons, 2017; Persson et al., 2018).

To maximize the performance of the individual chromatography step, the column size, flow rates and sequential procedure has to be selected. Parameter optimization based on mathematical models has proven to be the most efficient technique for this purpose. This has been done for capture (Baur et al., 2018; Gomis-Fons et al., 2020a, 2021; Klatt et al., 2000; Ng et al., 2012; Sellberg et al., 2018) and for other important steps (Borg et al., 2014; Saleh et al., 2020; Sellberg et al., 2017).

**Example 2.** *Continuous capture chromatography*

*Orbit controllers for different PCC processes has been developed and here is a more detailed presentation of a version configured on ÄKTA pure setup* (Gomis-Fons et al., 2020a). *The PCC configuration is seen in Fig. 8 where the sample pump continuously feed one column, in the figure the column 1. The flow through passes a set of versatile valves, a second UV detector and the outlet valve, and finally enter column 2. The flow-through of column 2 goes to waste. The third column is eluted by the A pump and passes the detector train before it is diluted to low pH by B pump and parked in the viral inactivation position. By simultaneously switching the loop valve and the three versatile values the three columns change mode of operation, the column 2 becomes the loading column followed by column 3, and column 1 is the one eluted.*

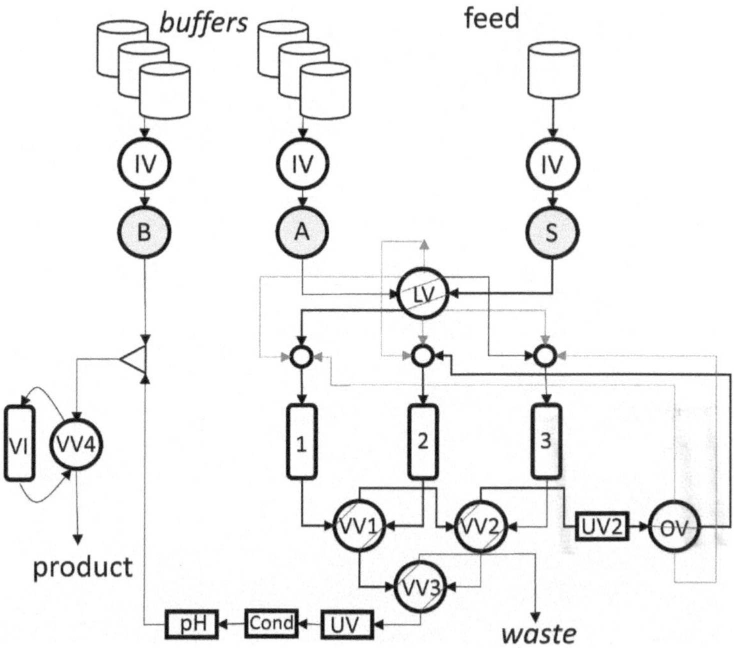


**Fig. 8** The general configuration of three column PCC on one experimental setup.

The introduction of continuous chromatography results in processes configured on multiple setups, because of parallel operation of the separation steps. In the example below the PCC-setup in the example above is complemented with a setup with two purification steps, two ion exchangers. Studies with a third parallel setup for a UFDF-step has also been performed. The automation of a multiple setup system can be structured in two different ways, centralized or distributed. Each experimental setup is controlled by a local Orbit controller. In the centralized version the complete automation is developed in one Orbit controller which sends control actions to the local Orbit clients, in a master-slave configuration. In the distributed version the automation of the local setup is done in the local Orbit controller. All local Orbit controllers interact with each other through handshaking at synchronization points at given positions in the automation procedures, see Fig. 9. Both versions have been studied but the distributed automation paradigm dominated in the examples presented here.

**Example 3.** *Continuous downstream processing of antibody*

*An integrated continuous downstream process for antibody purification based on PCC capture is illustrated in Fig. 10* (Gomis-Fons et al., 2020a). *The process uses the two basic configurations discussed above, the PCC implementation and the*

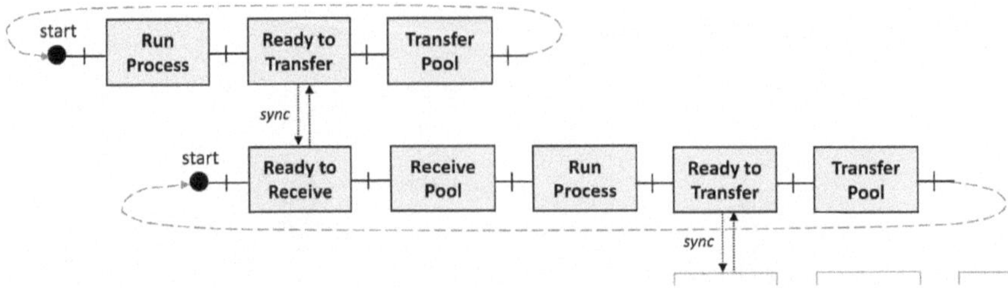


**Fig. 9** Synchronization between multiple local Orbit controllers in a distributed automation system.

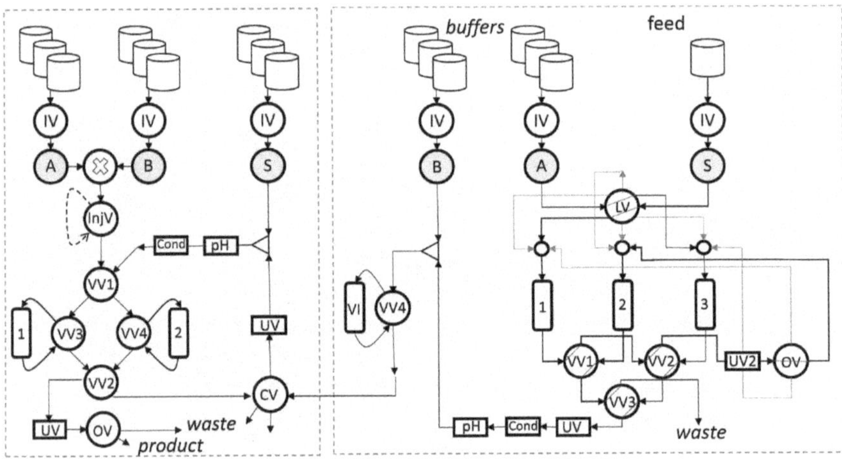


**Fig. 10** The general configuration of continuous downstream process for antibody purification in Example 3.

*sequential downstream process configuration. These two processes are configured on two different setups with their one orbit controllers. These orbit controllers communicate over the net to synchronize the processing. In this particular case it is done by handshaking at the specific position where a pool from the PCC system is delivered to the purification system.*

*The startup sequence of the process over the first 18h is seen in Fig. 11, which correspond to 6½ PCC switched (about 2 complete cycles). Each capture pool is parked for viral inactivation before it is loaded on the cation exchanger. The elution profiles in the purification process is seen below in Fig. 11. The cation exchanger is eluted and diluted in-line for direct loading of the flow-through anion exchanger. The dilution and the increased flow rate in the anion exchanger are the reasons the product peaks are smaller compared to cation exchanger pools.*

In the examples above a continuous downstream process for antibodies was presented. These processes have a general character as platform

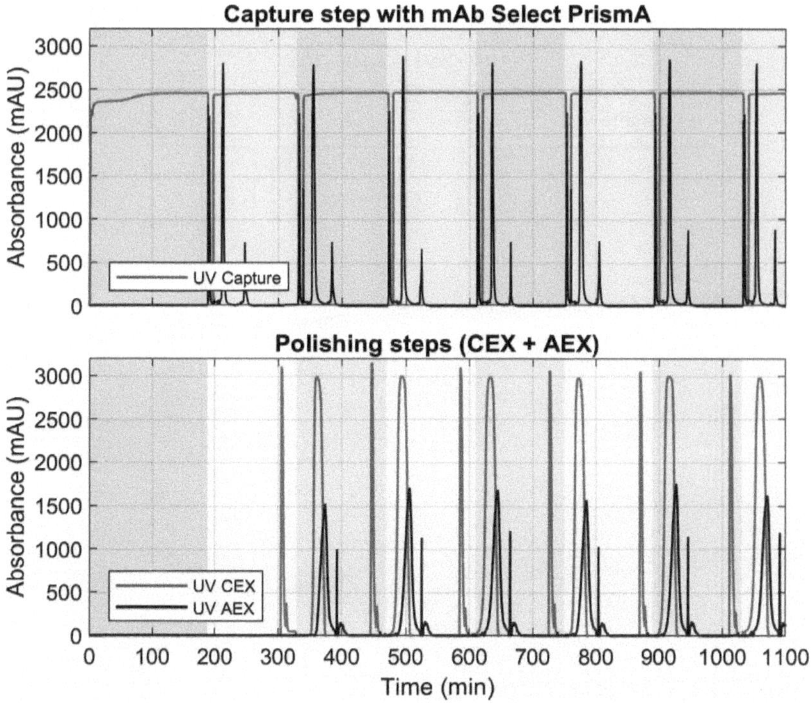


**Fig. 11** The chromatograms of continuous downstream process for antibody purification in Example 3.

processes and can be used or at least modified for purification of many different monoclonal antibodies. For other therapeutic proteins this is not the case. These downstream processes are often unique and tailor-made for the protein in question. One such unique process, for a fusion protein, was presented in Example 1. Another example of a downstream process for production of a therapeutic protein is presented in the next example. The downstream process was first developed for batch production, then modified into an integrated downstream process (Löfgren et al., 2018), and finally operated in full continuous downstream mode (Löfgren et al., 2021).

**Example 4.** *Continuous downstream processing of a protein*

*A therapeutic protein is purified in three step downstream process* (Löfgren et al., 2018). *The first step is an anion exchanger, for capture, followed by viral inactivation for one hour and the last step, for polishing, is a hydrophobic interaction column. The three steps was integrated and automated using the methodology discussed above. The complete chromatogram from one cycle is seen in Fig. 12.*

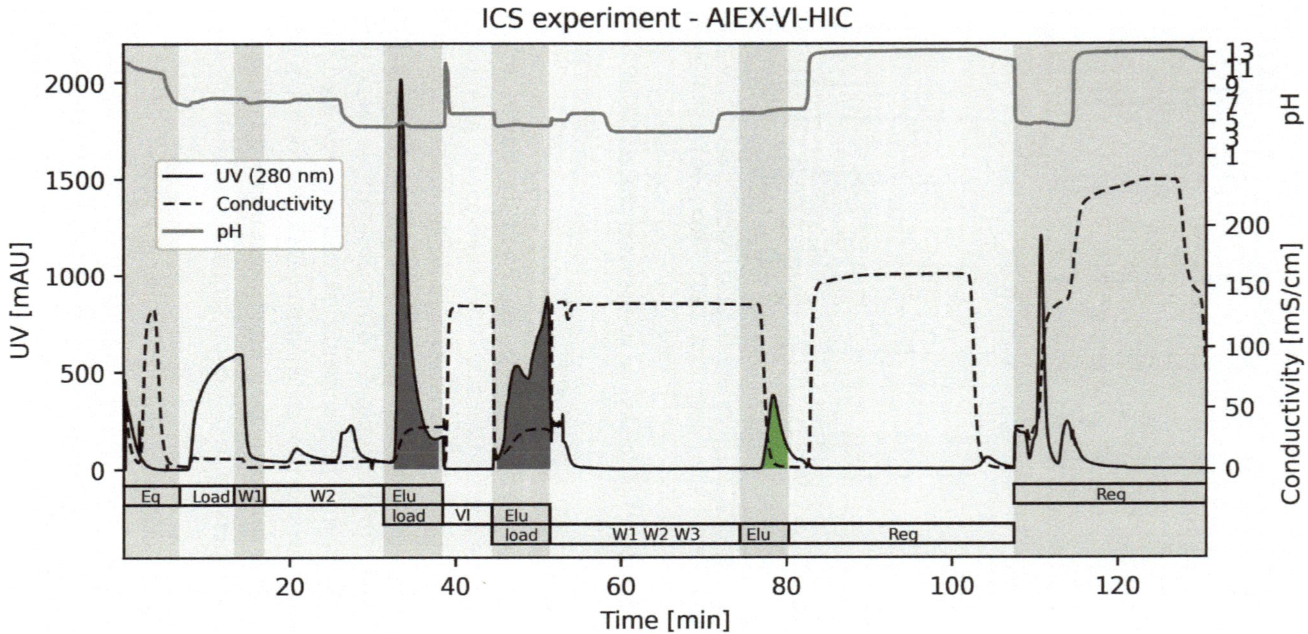


**Fig. 12** The complete chromatogram for the three step, ion exchange step with the pool at 110–130, viral inactivation pool at 150–170 and finally the hydrophobic interaction pool at 300–320, followed by cleaning procedures.

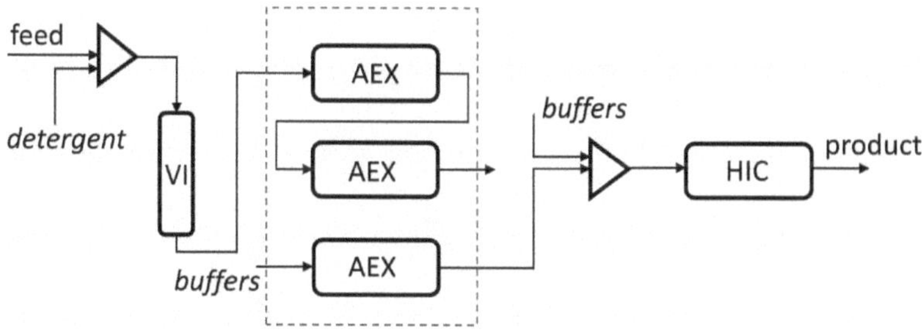


**Fig. 13** The continuous downstream process in Example 4.

*The integrated three step downstream process was turned into a continuous downstream process based on a PCC capture configuration with a continuous vital inactivation reactor before the PCC and a periodic HIC polishing step after the capture step, Fig. 13* (Löfgren et al., 2021). *The continuous viral inactivation was a detergent-based inactivation* (Martins et al., 2019) *to avoid low pH in the process.*

## 5. End-to-end production with continuous bioprocessing

Continuous biomanufacturing has got a lot of attention the last years and large efforts have been made to develop novel processing units and integrated continuous processes. Continuous production is often based on continuous upstream process based on perfusion (Godawat et al., 2015; Gomis-Fons et al., 2020b). The bioreactor operates at steady-state for a long time, with a membrane configuration to hold back cells and let the liquid with proteins pass. The perfusion system generates a continuous flow that changes slightly over time, except for the startup phase. The composition is also changing depending on the conditions in the bioreactor. The time scale in the bioreactor is slow compared to downstream. The downstream processes discussed above has an overall residence time of about 4–8 h while the bioreactor has residence time up to 24 h. This means that changes in the upstream systems will be seen as slow or almost constant from a cycle-to-cycle perspective by the downstream process.

To show the scalability of the methodology two antibody production examples are discussed below. The first example is the simplest and smallest complete continuous bioprocess studied. It is based on a 200 mL perfusion system with a continuous downstream process on one setup, even thou it was based on 1 mL prepacked columns, it had overcapacity. The second example is a scaled-up version to pilot-scale with a 30 L perfusion system.

Scaling of chromatography columns are quite straight forward (Hansen, 2017; Heuer et al., 1996). It is convenient to scale the sequential procedure in column volume and flow rate in residence time. This means that the design and operation of the column is scaled by its size. In an integrated synchronized sequence of columns the pool from the previous step is loaded directly to the next step. This creates two integration constraints; a capacity constraint and a flow rate constraint. This is discussed in Andersson et al. (2017) and Löfgren et al. (2019). The optimization of a typical column sequence connected to a continuous upstream process generates multiple designs, depending on the minimization of the residence time for the product of the column sizes.

**Example 5.** *Continuous antibody biomanufacturing in small-scale*

*A complete end-to-end biomanufacturing process was developed by integrating a small-scale perfusion system with a small-scale downstream process on one experimental setup* (Gomis-Fons et al., 2020b), *illustrated in Fig. 14. The downstream process consists of two capture columns that run in parallel, allowing the continuous loading of one column and the elution of the other. After the parallel capture step, a conventional antibody platform is integrated, with low pH based viral inactivation and two ion exchangers for purification. Between the two systems, upstream and downstream, a balance tank was needed. There are two reasons for this design. The first is that the permeate pump in the perfusion system is not designed for the loading of packed bed columns which forces the addition of an intermediate tank to give the possibility to use high pressure pump instead. The benefit with this design is that it gives the downstream process a small window of freedom for trouble-shooting and reconfiguration between the different cycles, if needed. The process illustrated in Fig. 14 can be configured in principle as Fig. 5, where the parallel capture and the cation exchanger are odd steps and the viral inactivation and the anion exchanger are odd.*

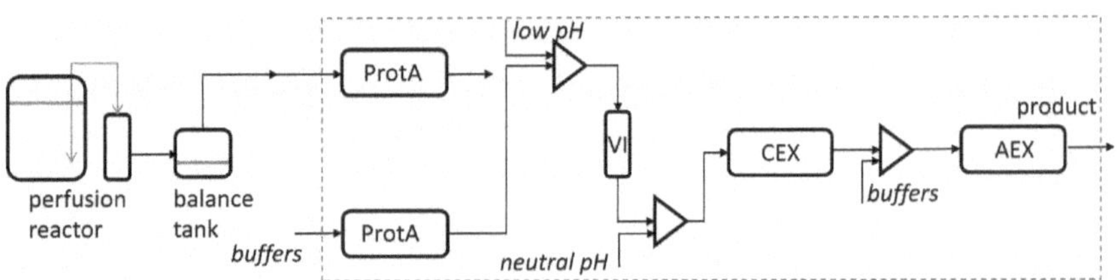


**Fig. 14** The process diagram for a complete continuous biomanufacturing system.

To illustrate the scalability of the methodology the second example is based on a continuous bioprocess for the production of antibodies similar to the previous. The capture is a continuous PCC setup and the downstream process is configured as in Example 3. The complete automated bioprocess was first operated in lab-scale based on a 200 mL bioreactor. Then it was scaled up 150 times to 30 L bioreactor connected to the same downstream process and automation system. It was only the sizes of the chromatography columns that was adjusted to the nominal perfusion flow rate and nominal titer. Note that the automation of the whole downstream process was scaled according to the individual column sizes and loading.

**Example 6.** *Scale-up of end-to-end continuous biomanufacturing of monoclonal antibody*

*A complete end-to-end integrated continuous biomanufacturing process for monoclonal antibody was developed, based on perfusion upstream process with a continuous downstream process. This process was both implemented and operated in lab-scale and then scaled up 150 times to pilot scale. The downstream process was design for pH sensitive antibodies operated at only pH 5.5 and higher. A calcium dependent Protein A ligand was used in the capture step allowing control of the elution by salt* (Scheffel and Hober, 2021). *It also means that the viral inactivation needs to be done by detergent instead of low pH* (Martins et al., 2019). *The process flow sheet is seen in Fig. 15.*

*The three-column PCC was configured on a pcc setup and the purification was configured on a pure setup. Three cycles, and nine pcc switches, is seen in Fig. 16. In this case three capture pools was collected in one hold-up tank before the viral inactivation started. After one hour the inactivation pool is loaded on the cation exchanger.*

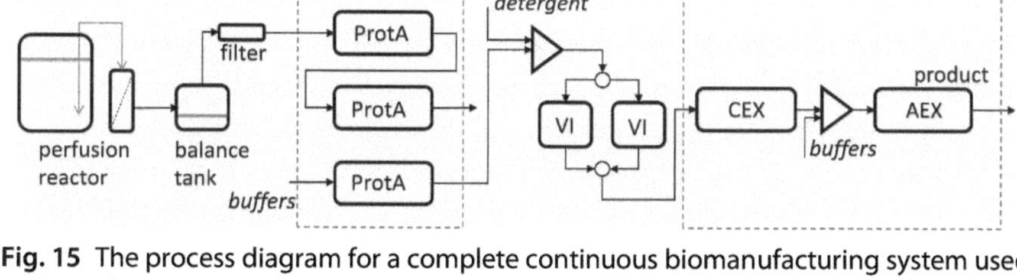


**Fig. 15** The process diagram for a complete continuous biomanufacturing system used in Example 6.

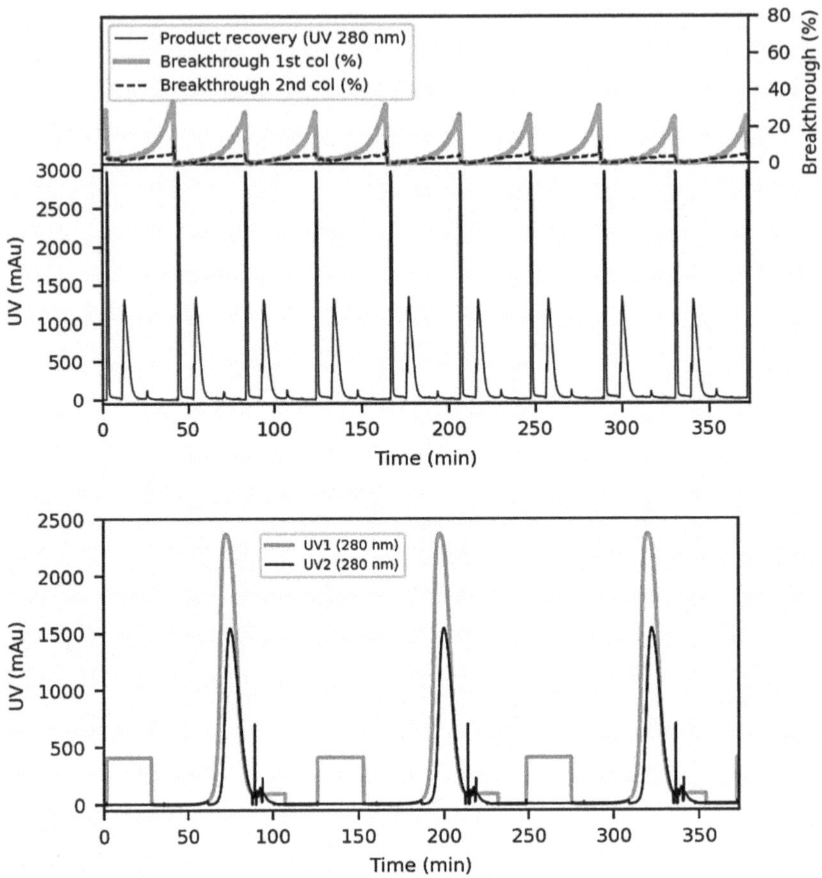


**Fig. 16** The chromatograms of continuous downstream process for antibody purification in Example 6.

## 6. Control of continuous downstream processes

The operation of a continuous downstream process connected to a continuous upstream process, like a perfusion system, needs to be controlled to compensate for changing conditions. During long-term operation the conditions in the upstream process changes, which means that the feed flow rate and composition changes. Compared to the dynamics in the downstream process, the upstream changes are slow or very slow. Long term operation and high number of separation cycles also induce changing properties in the downstream processing steps, like decreased capacity. This means that it is hard to run the continuous downstream process at its nominal operating conditions without sacrificing performance and quality. Therefore, there is a need for real-time control that compensate for disturbances and deviations (Feidl et al., 2020; Rathore et al., 2021; Steinebach et al., 2017; Vogg et al., 2018). Important control problems are the following:

1. Loading control of capture step for optimal operation of the capture step. Note this also scale all pools for the other separation steps, if they run synchronously.
2. Separation and retention control of purification steps for the removal of important impurities.
3. Pooling control of all steps for the selection of cut times for purity.
4. Monitoring of quality attributes to guarantee quality.

Traditional loading control of capture steps utilize the measurement of a small amount of breakthrough of the product. This control system is very robust and can handle many different disturbances in the process, from feed changes to resin degradation. The drawback is that the breakthrough of the product can be very hard to detect, particular in upstream systems with low or very low titer and with large amounts of contaminants. This was the case for the case study discussed in Example 4. An alternative control system that minimizes product losses is presented below.

**Example 7.** *Advanced loading control*

*The continuous downstream process for a therapeutic protein is presented in Example 3* (Löfgren et al., 2021). *Based on the low concentration of the target comped to impurities, together with high requirements an advanced loading control was developed. The traditional UV-based breakthrough control was not suitable. Instead, the resulting product pool from the polishing step was used as measurement in a loading controller that uses the PCC cycle time are control signal, see the block diagram in Fig. 17. As a reference signal is the nominal size of the product peek. Note that a controller like this is a batch-to-batch controller or iterative learning control* (Longman, 2000), *where the previous batch result, $y_{k-1}$, is used in the adjustment of the conditions for the next batch, $u_k$.*

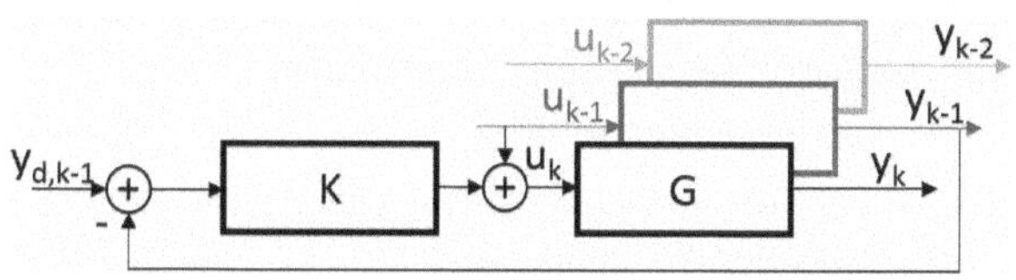


**Fig. 17** Block diagram for the batch-to-batch loading controller.

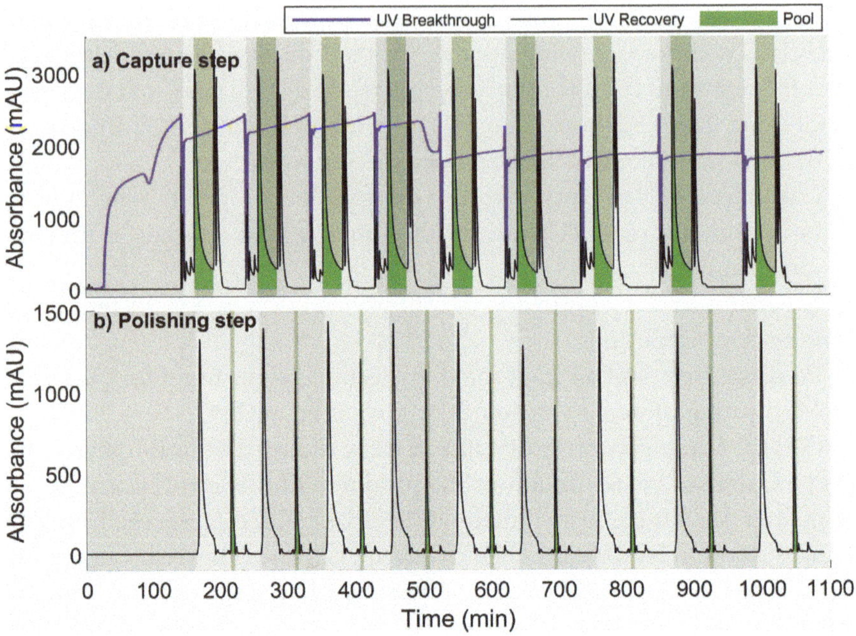


**Fig. 18** The chromatograms of continuous downstream process in Example 7. Note the disturbance in feed concentration at switch 4.

*The behavior of the controlled continuous downstream process is seen in the chromatograms in Fig. 18. It illustrate the startup the process and the UV detector signal in both the PCC based capture setup and the poliching step. Note that the small peek in the polishing step chromatogram is the product.*

*A distubance in the feed concentration enters at switch 4, about at 500 min, in the PCC setup. This disturbance is seen in the product peek first at 700 min. The performance of the batch-to-batch controller is seen in Fig. 19. The controller recover to the desired value in one batch.*

In the purification steps it is important to control the purity but also try to keep up the performance of the step. During long-term operation the condition in the feed and in the buffers changes, resulting in changes in retention and therefore resolution causing possible change in purity. It is therefore interesting to control the retention in the purification steps to guarantee both quality and performance during purification.

**Example 8.** *Advanced separation control*

*Two proteins are separated, one target and one product related impurity, by a gradient based cation exchange chromatography step. A multivariable batch-to-batch controller, that uses retention times for the two peaks as measurements and the amount*

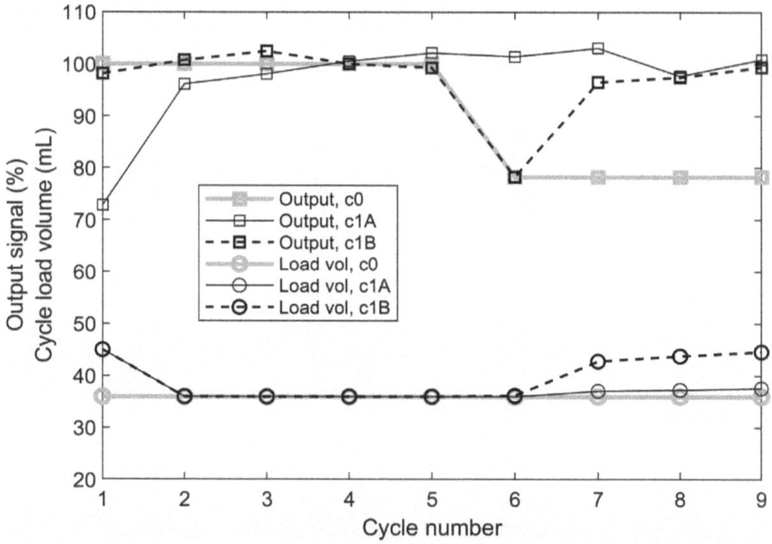


**Fig. 19** The output signal (pool size) and the cycle length (loading time) in Example 7. Note that the disturbance at batch 6 is recovered directly in batch 7.

*of elution buffer at the start and the end of the gradient as control signals, is used for separation control, see Fig. 17* (Espinoza et al., 2022). *The controller performance for nine cycles is seen in Fig. 20. The chromatogram for cycle 2 to 4 as also seen. At cycle 3 the pH changes in the buffers from 6.8 to 7.5. The controller can keep the separation step at desired retention times by slightly changing the gradient.*

All separations steps have some kind of pooling control in order to direct a part of the outflow in a desired direction, product pool, and the rest to waste. This pooling control can be straightforward based on time or volume. More advanced control are based on detector signals for the location of the pool, for instance UV-based pooling.

**Example 9.** *Advanced pooling control*

*In the small-scale end-to-end continuous bioprocess in Example 2, a advanced pooling control was used* (Gomis-Fons et al., 2020b). *The pooling controller was used to pool the cation exchanger product, pool the monomer antibody and reduce the amount of aggregate forms. The aggregates appear on the rear part of the chromatogram, see Fig. 21. The condition in the perfusion system changes and the result was that the amount of antibody loaded on the column changed a lot. In order to decrease product losses the UV-based cut points was scaled by the amount pooled from the previous step, in a model-based feed-forward controller.*

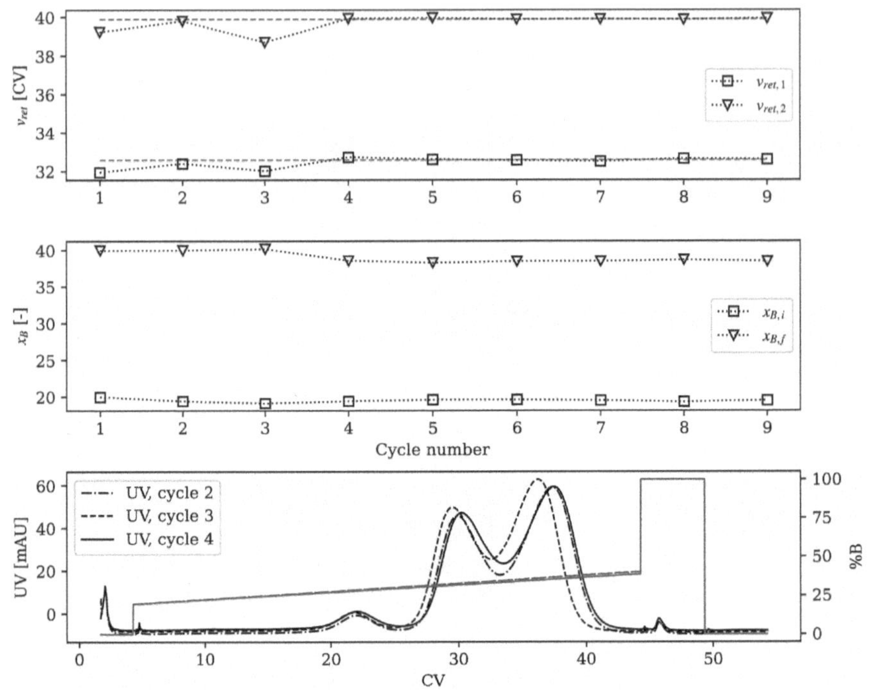


**Fig. 20** The chromatograms of continuous downstream process in.

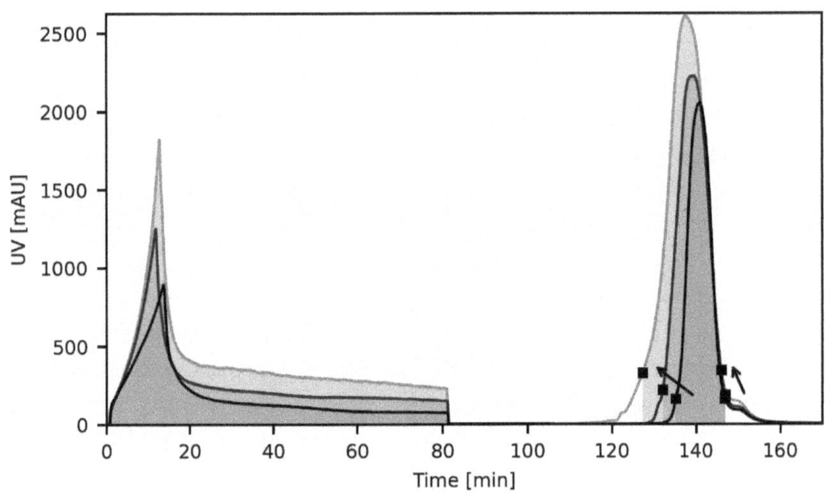


**Fig. 21** Advanced pooling control in Example 9 used to pool an ion exchange step in Example 2.

Integration and automation of analytical methods are important in continuous processing to monitor quality attributes in real time (Dagge et al., 2009). These methods often needs sampling of the flow path to perform analysis of the composition, e.g. HPLC with advanced detectors, like MS. This online analysis can be time critical for the use of downstream control or not so critical used for the monitoring of process characteristics. Orbit can communicate with HPLC systems, which can be integrated into any of the processes presented here.

**Example 10.** *Integrated online analytics*

*The integrated downstream process for a therapeutic protein, presented in Example 1* (Gomis-Fons et al., *2019*)*, was integrated with an HPLC for online analytics* (Tallvod et al., 2022). *After each step the pool was sampled and pumped to the injection valve of the HPLC. This was performed by the process setup controller. The process controller then synchronized with the HPLC controller. The HPLC controller performs the analysis procedure and when it is done it is back to waiting position ready for a new analysis* (Fig. 22).

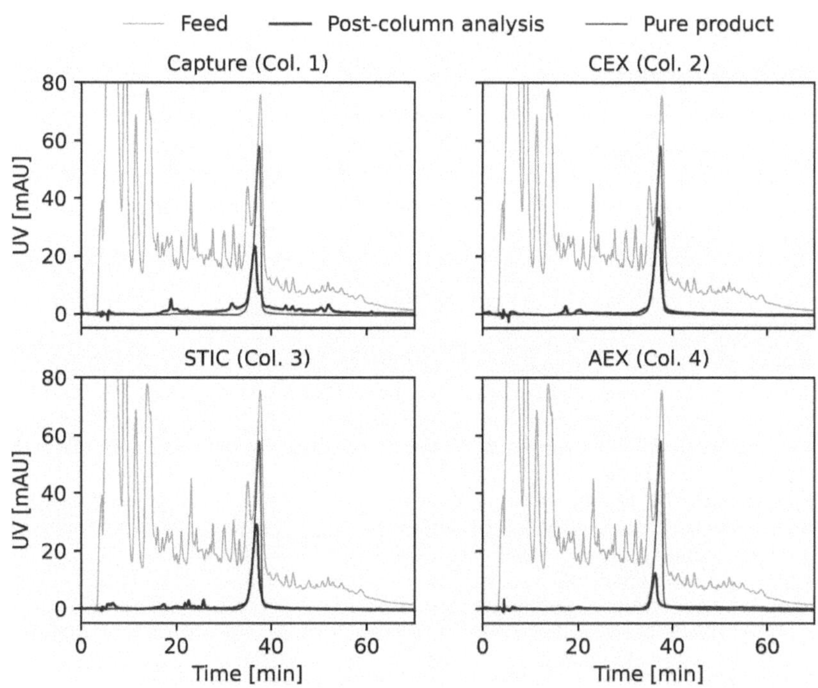


**Fig. 22** The HPLC chromatogram for analysis of the pools from the different chromatography steps in Example 1.

## 7. Summary

This chapter presents a smart platform for development of automated integrated continuous downstream processes. The platform is based on using common available equipment and reconfigure them for advanced downstream processing. The process is automated by an external supervisory controller, communicating with the local equipment control system. The supervisory controller, called Orbit, is implemented in an open, flexible, and extendable environment in Python, giving the user support for advanced process development. Orbit give support for integration of multiple chromatography columns on one setup, operate downstream processes on multiple parallel setups, integrated online analytics, use advanced feedback control and batch-to-batch control. This functionality has been presented in 10 examples. The smart platform use minimal additional resources and changes in the laboratory infrastructure. The platform has successful been used in number of industrial case studies, particular in early drug and process development.

## Acknowledgments

The authors thank Daniel Espinoza and Simon Tallvod for help with the manuscript. This work is financially supported by Swedish Innovation Agency, Vinnova, under Grant 2019-05314 (AutoPilot project) and Grant 2016-0518 (Competence Centre for Advanced BioProduction by Continuous Processing, AdBIOPRO), and the support from industrial partners BioInvent, Cytiva, Modelon, Novo Nordisk and Sobi.

## References

Andersson N, Löfgren A, Olofsson M, SellBerg A, Nilsson B: Design and control of integrated chromatography columns sequences, *Biotechnol Prog* 33:923–930, 2017.

Baur D, Angarita M, Müller-Späth T, Steinebach F, Morbidelli M: Comparison of batch and continuous multi-column protein A capture processes by optimal design, *Biotechnol J* 11(7):920–931, 2016a.

Baur D, Angarita M, Muller-Spath T, Morbidelli M: Optimal model-based design of the twin-column CaptureSMB process improves capacity utilization and productivity in protein A affinity capture, *Biotechnol J* 11(1):135–145, 2016b.

Baur D, Angelo JM, Chollangi S, et al.: Model assisted comparison of Protein A resins and multi-column chromatography for capture processes, *J Biotechnol* 285:64–73, 2018.

Borg N, Brodsky Y, Moscariello J, et al.: Modeling and robust pooling design of a preparative cation-exchange chromatography step for purification of monoclonal antibody monomer from aggregates, *J Chromatogr A* 1359:170–181, 2014.

Dagge L, Harr K, Paul M, Schnedl G: Classification of process analysis: offline—atline—online—inline, *Cement Int* 7(5):72–81, 2009.

Espinoza D, Andersson N, Nilsson B: In-silico formulation of iterative learning control for chromatographic purification of biopharmaceuticals, In Proceedings of the 32th European Symposium on Computer Aided Process Engineering. 2022.

Farid SS: Process economics of industrial monoclonal antibody manufacture, *J Chromatogr B* 848(1):8–18, 2007.

Feidl F, Vogg S, Wolf M, et al.: Process-wide control and automation of an integrated continuous manufacturing platform for antibodies, *Biotechnol Bioeng* 117(5): 1367–1380, 2020.

Godawat R, Brower K, Jain S, Konstantinov K, Riske F, Warikoo V: Periodic counter-current chromatography—design and operational considerations for integrated and continuous purification of proteins, *Biotechnol J* 7(12):1496–1508, 2012.

Godawat R, Konstantinov K, Rohani M, Warikoo V: End-to-end integrated fully continuous production of recombinant monoclonal antibodies, *J Biotechnol* 213 (Supplement C):13–19, 2015.

Gomis-Fons J: *Simulation, optimization and implementation of a twin-column MCSGP process for the purification of Liraglutide*, MSc thesis, Sweden, 2017, Lund University.

Gomis-Fons J, Löfgren A, Andersson N, Nilsson B, Berghard L, Wood S: Integration of a complete downstream process for the automated lab-scale production of a recombinant protein, *J Biotechnol* 301(2019):45–51, 2019.

Gomis-Fons J, Andersson N, Nilsson B: Optimization study on periodic counter-current chromatography integrated in a monoclonal antibody downstream process, *J Chrom A* 1621: 461055, 2020a.

Gomis-Fons J, Schwarz H, Zhang L, et al.: Model-based design and control of a small-scale integrated continuous end-to-end mAb platform, *Biotechnol Progr* 36(1), 2020b.

Gomis-Fons J, Yamanee-Nolin M, Andersson N, Nilsson B: Optimal loading flow rate trajectory in monoclonal antibody capture chromatography, *J Chrom A* 1635(2020): 461760, 2021.

Hansen EB: Chromatographic scale-up on a volume basis, In Staby A, Rathore AS, Ahuja S, editors: *Preparative chromatography for separation of proteins*, 2017, John Wiley & Sons, Inc.

Heuer C, Hugo P, Mann G, Seidel-Morgenstern A: Scale up in preparative chromatography, *J Chromatogr A* 752(1):19–29, 1996.

Kesik-Brodacka M: Progress in biopharmaceutical development, *Biotechnol Appl Biochem* 65(3):306–322, 2018. https://doi.org/10.1002/bab.1617.

Klatt K-U, Hanisch F, Dünnebier G, Engell S: Model-based optimization and control of chromatographic processes, *Comput Chem Eng* 24(2):1119–1126, 2000.

Konstantinov KB, Cooney CL: White paper on continuous bioprocessing May 20–21 2014 continuous manufacturing symposium, *J Pharm Sci* 104(3):813–820, 2015.

Löfgren A, Andersson N, Sellberg A, Nilsson B, Löfgren M, Woods S: Designing an autonomous integrated downstream sequence from a batch separation process—an industrial case study, *Biotechnol J* 2018:1700691, 2018.

Löfgren A, Yamanee-Nolin M, Tallvod S, Gomis Fons J, Andersson N, Nilsson B: Optimization of integrated chromatography sequences for purification of biopharmaceuticals, *Biotechnol Prog* 35(6): e2871, 2019.

Löfgren A, Gomis-Fons J, Andersson N, Nilsson B, Berghard L, Lagerqvist Hägglund C: An integrated continuous downstream process with real-time control: a case study with periodic counter-current chromatography and continuous virus inactivation, *Biotechnol Bioeng*, 2021.

Longman RW: Iterative learning control and repetitive control for engineering practice, *Int J Control* 73(10):930–954, 2000.

Martins DL, Sencar J, Hammerschmidt N, et al.: Continuous solvent/detergent virus inactivation using a packed-bed reactor, *Biotechnol J* 14(8):1800646, 2019.

Moreno-González M, Keulen D, Gomis-Fons J, Gomez GL, Nilsson B, Ottens M: Continuous adsorption in food industry: the recovery of sinapic acid from rapeseed meal extract, *J Sep Pur* 254: 117403, 2021.

Ng CKS, Osuna-Sanchez H, Valéry E, Sørensen E, Bracewell DG: Design of high productivity antibody capture by protein A chromatography using an integrated experimental and modeling approach, *J Chromatogr B* 899(Supplement C):116–126, 2012.

Persson O, Andersson N, Nilsson B: Design of two-column batch-to-batch recirculation to enhanced performance in ion-exchange chromatography, *J Chrom A* 1531: 112–121, 2018.

Rathore AS, Nikita S, Thakur G, Deore N: Challenges in process control for continuous processing for production of monoclonal antibody products, *Curr Opin Chem Eng* 31:100671, 2021.

Riske F, Ransohoff T: Development of continuous capture steps in bioprocess applications, In Staby A, Rathore AS, Ahuja S, editors: *Preparative chromatography for separation of proteins*, 2017, John Wiley & Sons, Inc.

Saleh D, Wang G, Müller B, et al.: Straightforward method for calibration of mechanistic cation exchange chromatography models for industrial applications, *Biotechnol Progr* 36(4): e2984, 2020.

Scheffel J, Hober S: Highly selective Protein A resin allows for mild sodium chloride-mediated elution of antibodies, *J Chromatogr A* 1637:461843, 2021.

Sellberg A, Holmqvist A, Magnusson F, Andersson C, Nilsson B: Discretized multi-level trajectory: a proof-of-concept demonstration, *J Chrom A* 1481:73–81, 2017.

Sellberg A, Nolin M, Löfgren A, Andersson N, Nilsson B: In *Multi-flowrate optimization of the loading phase of a preparative chromatography separation*, Proceedings of ESCAPE28 2018, Graz, Austria. 2018.

Shi C, Zhang Q-L, Jiao B, et al.: Process development and optimization of continuous capture with three-column periodic counter-current chromatography, *Biotechnol Bioeng* 118(9):3313–3322, 2021.

Shukla AA, Thömmes J: Recent advances in large-scale production of monoclonal antibodies and related proteins, *Trends Biotechnol* 28(5):253–261, 2010.

Shukla AA, Wolfe LS, Mostafa SS, Norman C: Evolving trends in mAb production processes, *Bioeng Transl Med* 2(1):58–69, 2017. https://doi.org/10.1002/btm2.10061.

Steinebach F, Ulmer N, Wolf M, et al.: Design and operation of a continuous integrated monoclonal antibody production process, *Biotechnol Progr* 33(5):1303–1313, 2017.

Tallvod S, Yamanee-Nolin M, Gomis-Fons J, Andersson N, Nilsson B: A novel process design for automated quality analysis in an integrated biopharmaceutical platform, In Proceedings of the 32nd European Symposium on Computer Aided Process Engineering. 2022.

Vogg S, Müller-Späth T, Morbidelli M: Current status and future challenges in continuous biochromatography, *Curr Opin Chem Eng* 22:138–144, 2018.

Walther J, Godawat R, Hwang C, Abe Y, Sinclair A, Konstantinov K: The business impact of an integrated continuous biomanufacturing platform for recombinant protein production, *J Biotechnol* 213:3–12, 2015.

Zydney AL: Perspectives on integrated continuous bioprocessing—opportunities and challenges, *Curr Opin Chem Eng* 10(Supplement C):8–13, 2015.

CHAPTER SIX

# Fill-Finish: Large-scale manufacturing considerations

**Silvia Cieri***
F. Hoffmann-La Roche AG, Dept. Global Manufacturing Science and Technology, Basel, Switzerland
*Corresponding author: e-mail address: silvia.cieri@roche.com

## Contents



*Advances in Chemical Engineering*, Volume 59
ISSN 0065-2377
https://doi.org/10.1016/bs.ache.2022.03.005

## Abstract

Fill-Finish operations, including all the processes and activities that get the pharmaceutical component ready for distribution and commercialization as a Drug Product (DP), cover a significant portion of the whole biopharmaceutical manufacturing, in terms of both process complexity and processing costs. In this chapter, the traditional unit operations that are in place from the acceptance of the drug substance to the final packaging are presented and discussed highlighting the critical requirements in terms of sterility, safety and regulatory aspects. A typical flowchart is discussed, together with the available alternatives for the equipment deputed to each operation, with their pros and cons. After the main concepts underlying the Fill-Finish section are presented, the discussion is shifted toward the trends that this section of the biopharmaceutical manufacturing is experiencing. The road toward a personalized medicine taken in the last years by the (bio)pharmaceutical companies is leading to a radical change in the paradigm, translated in the miniaturization of the equipment and the pursuit of process versatility, production on demand and fast change-over. These aspects are discussed herein, stressing the interdisciplinarity of the competences required to reach a comprehensive solution.

## Abbreviations

**ASTM** American Society for Testing and Materials
**AVI** automatic visual inspection
**CCI** container closure integrity
**CG&T** cell & gene therapies
**DS** drug substance
**DP** drug product
**EMA** European Medicine Agency
**FDA** Food and Drug Administration
**F/T** freeze and thaw
**GMP** good manufacturing practices
**RABS** restricted area barrier system
**SAL** sterility assurance level
**SS** stainless steel
**SU** single use
**USP** United States Pharmacopeia
**WHO** World Health Organization

## 1. Introduction

This chapter describes unit operations and components used in the Fill-Finish manufacturing of a sterile product.

The manufacture of a sterile product is subject to special requirements in order to minimize risks of microbiological, particulate and pyrogenic contamination.

Manufacturing operations are divided into two categories:

- products that are terminally sterilized
- products that are conducted aseptically at some or all stages (focus of this chapter)

Fill-Finish operations are the series of steps after the drug substance preparation (upstream and downstream) that include formulation, aseptic filling, stoppering, inspection and secondary packaging. Additional steps may be added as required by the molecule.

Acceptance of Drug substance is the starting point for Fill-Finish operations.

Drug substances may come under different forms, usually as frozen solutions or solid powders. Based on the drug substance presentation, the handling of the substance will require different unit operations and area classification. For example, frozen solutions will require a validated process for thawing while powders will require a specific compounding step for further processing in a solution phase. Handling of powder should be carefully considered as, based on the density of the product, personnel needs to be protected by exposure to the risk of contact/inhalation of powder.

## 2. cGMP and pharmacopeia

The manufacturing process of each drug should undergo approval by regulators, the minimum set of requirements to be satisfied are described in the Current Good Manufacturing Practices (cGMPs), which are the set of production standards that have been embraced by regulators, retailers and consumers in the food and drug industries.

The cGMP regulations for drugs contain minimum requirements for the methods, facilities, and controls used in manufacturing, processing, and packing of a drug product. The regulations make sure that a product is safe for use, and that it has the ingredients and strength it claims to have.

In addition to the cGMP, a legally binding collection of standards and quality specifications for medicine is collected in the Pharmacopeia. Within the pharmacopoeia, a quality specification is a set of appropriate tests that will confirm the identity and purity of the product, as certain the strength (or amount) of the active substance and, when needed, the performance characteristics. Pharmacopeia are existing for each region/country in which the manufacturer is intending to distribute the drugs.

## 3. Regulatory landscape

As mentioned in Section 2, the approval of each drug must undergo a step of review and acceptance by regulators. Pharmaceutical Regulators are country wise or region wise responsible for authorizing the marketing distribution of new medicines.

The Food and Drugs Administration (FDA) is the Drug Regulatory Authority responsible for review, approval, and post approval compliance of all the drugs being marketed in the United States.

The European Medicine Agency (EMA) is absolving comparable role for the European region. An overview of European regulators by countries is provided in The European Regulatory System (2016), a consistent approach to medicines regulation, 2016.

On top of national/region-based regulators, listed in Global Regulatory Authority Websites (n.d.), many international and multinational organizations are active in the effort of maintaining alignment and standard across the different regulations.

## 4. General considerations on the manufacturing plant for Fill-Finish operations of an aseptic filled sterile product

The manufacturing of an aseptic filled sterile product must be carried out in a facility that is respecting the following basic criteria. These entire requirements are established to minimize the level of contamination and provide the highest quality standards.

### 4.1 Facility design

The manufacture of sterile products should be carried out in clean areas to which entry should be through airlocks for personnel and/or for equipment and materials. Clean areas for the manufacture of sterile products are classified according to the required characteristics of the environment. Each manufacturing operation requires an appropriate environmental cleanliness level in the operational state in order to minimize the risks of particulate or microbial contamination of the product or materials being handled.

The flow of materials and personnel through the building or facilities should be designed to prevent mix-ups or contamination.

## 4.2 Monitoring program

When aseptic operations are performed, environmental monitoring should be frequent using methods such as settle plates, volumetric air and surface. Surfaces and personnel should be monitored after critical operations. Additional microbiological monitoring is also required outside production operations, e.g., after validation of systems, cleaning and sanitization. Personnel periodic qualification is required for who working in critical operations as aseptic filling and visual inspection.

## 4.3 Personnel

All personnel employed in clean areas and, generally, in the manufacturing of a sterile product should receive regular training in disciplines relevant to the correct manufacture of sterile products. This training should include reference to hygiene and to the basic elements of microbiology.

## 4.4 Utilities

All utilities that could affect product quality (e.g., steam, gas, compressed air, heating, ventilation, and air conditioning) should be qualified and appropriately monitored and action should be taken when pre-establish limits are exceeded.

## 4.5 Water

Water used in the manufacture of sterile products should be demonstrated to be suitable for its intended use. Where water used in the process is treated by the manufacturer to achieve a defined quality, the treatment process should be validated and monitored with appropriate action limits.

# 5. Fill-Finish process overview

When manufacturing a sterile product, precautions to minimize contamination should be taken during all processing stages including the stages before sterilization.

A comprehensive plan and execution of validation activities and process simulation must be carried out to demonstrate robustness and repeatability of successful aseptic handling.

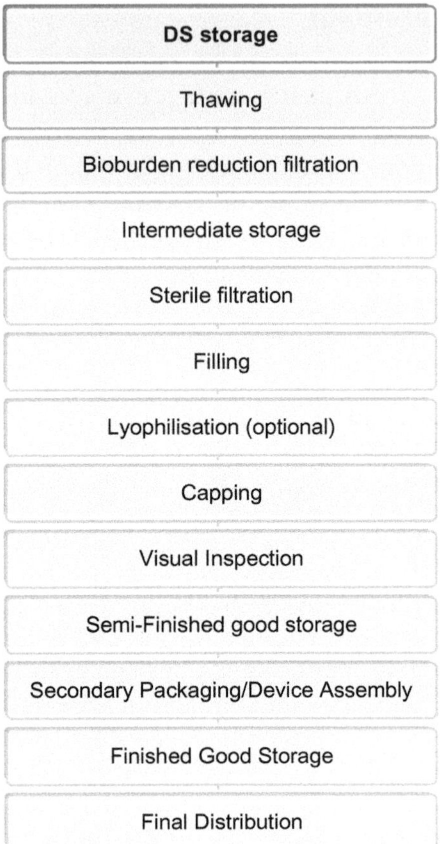


**Fig. 1** Process flow chart, Fill-Finish unit operations.

## 5.1 Process flowchart

The process flow chart presented in Fig. 1 is providing an overview of a common Fill-Finish operation set up for sterile products (aseptically produced). Steps may vary or been skipped due to the specific nature of the product in scope.

## 5.2 DS storage and delivery to DP site

When manufacturing a sterile product via aseptic procedures, the Drug Substance (DS) is usually formulated in liquid status and stored frozen to prevent product degradation, microbial growth, foam formation and product stress during shipment.

The shipment of the DS to the Drug Product (DP) site is an important step and the following requirement needs to be satisfied:

- product identity needs to be confirmed at the receiving site
- the shipping container must be technically compatible to both sites (DS and DP sites)
- temperature excursion over shipment needs to be avoided/limited and their product quality impact must be known/investigated
- integrity of the container over shipment must be granted through a validated procedure

Two families of storage container are vastly used for DS storage and shipping: cryovessels and single use bags. The selection of the most appropriate container is based on the product characteristics as highlighted in Table 1.

## 5.3 Freeze/thaw (F/T)

Upon DS delivery to the DP site, a thawing step is needed to be able to process the Drug Substance.

For biological products, the methodology of freezing/thawing may influence the stability of protein included in the DS formulation and its physic-chemical characteristics. Therefore, a freezing and thawing recipe (at a controlled rate), needs to be qualified demonstrating that the DS is homogeneous in a liquid status prior to transfer to a storage container (Pooling/Mixing step) and that the freezing was not leading to any protein aggregation.

**Table 1** Cryovessel, single use bag comparison for DS storage and shipping.

| | Cryovessel | Single use bag |
|---|---|---|
| Product volume | Big | Small |
| Shipping stress | Low fragility, robust solution | Higher fragility, the bag needs proper mechanical protection |
| Extractable | SS material, limited risk of product contamination | Bag materials and resistance to the product must be demonstrated |
| Cleaning | Cleaning Validation must be implemented for each product | Single Use component |
| Sustainability | Multiple shipments required for each product transfer (empty vessel return). Cleaning and sanitization required at each use | Bag needs to be decontaminated after use, high amount of waste (not recyclable material) |

The F/T recipe varies based on the container where the DS is stored.

- Cryovessel: recipe using silicone oil media are usually implemented
- Single-Use bag: a bath in water is normally foreseen

After completion of the thawing recipe, the solution is transferred to a different container and, in case the product is not fully used, the DS could be frozen again. The total number of F/T cycles, and the conditions that are anticipated for commercial production must be assessed for product quality impact prior to or concurrent with commercial-scale validation. These studies may be performed with material representative of the commercial process.

Additional studies to support microbial and chemical hold time over the different conditions to which the solution is exposed (e.g., frozen, cold, ambient), should be foreseen to guarantee product quality over time.

## 5.4 Filtration (bioburden reduction and sterile filtration)

After the completion of thawing of the Drug Substance, the solution may be transferred in a storage container or immediately filtered for bioburden reduction.

The levels of bacterial endotoxins in the finished product can be impacted by the bioburden and bacterial endotoxins in the components (i.e., active substance, excipients and containers), and by microbiological contaminants introduced during manufacture. To ensure an acceptable level of bacterial endotoxins in the finished product, the level of microbiological contaminants of the components should be minimal. Acceptance criteria for bioburden and, where relevant, bacterial endotoxins in components and bulk solutions should be specified and controlled along the manufacturing steps.

The bioburden reduction filtration and the sterile filtration are crucial for aseptically handled products. In accordance with EMA (Annex 1—Manufacture of Sterile Medicinal Products, 2008), if terminal sterilization is not applicable due to product sensitivity to temperature, the liquid product should be sterilized by filtration through a sterile, sterilizing grade filter and subsequently aseptically filled into a previously sterilized container.

Multiple filtration steps are usually needed to achieve this goal (filter train). The bioburden reduction filtration step is a pre-step for reducing microbial contaminants while sterile filtration is carried out as close as possible to the filling point. Regulatory expectations for sterilizing grade filters are outlined in the FDA Aseptic Processing Guideline.

Bioburden reduction and sterile filters have generally nominal pore size of 0.22 μm (or less), and demonstrated micro-organism retaining properties.

Such filters can remove most bacteria and molds, but not all viruses or mycoplasmas (different contamination prevention and clearance strategies are applied during Drug Substance processing to reduce possible introduction of viruses and mycoplasmas through DS into DP). The microbial retention by the membrane is based on the principle of size exclusion. The membrane pore must be smaller than the microorganism to be retained[1] (Steffen and Giglia, n.d.).

The integrity of the sterilized filter is verified before use and should be confirmed immediately after use by an appropriate method such as a bubble test. These tests confirm that the filter meets a defined specification for retention assurance and links the condition of filter operation to the validation of filter performance (FDA, 1999, 2016, n.d.).

The filter should not affect the product by removal of ingredients from it or by release of substances into it; testing on filter compatibility, absorption and leachables have to be considered and planned during product development and confirmed during process validation.

## 5.5 Pooling and mixing

Solution pooling is required when mixing multiple DS batches to achieve a desired volume.

During pooling a mixing step via agitation may or may not occur, agitation is instead required when mixing DS and buffer/excipient (e.g., compounding/dilution).

Agitation is controlled by mixers setting and design. In general, top- or center-mounted mixers are better suited for products that require aggressive or rapid blending. While bottom-mounted magnetic mixers are good for easy, gentle movement of product in your vessel (Fig. 2).

Moreover, when executing a pooling/mixing step the following aspects must be controlled:

- Homogeneity: no gradient in the solution. Homogeneity is defined using quality attribute(s), e.g., concentration, refractive index, osmolality and it needs to be controlled as part of qualification collecting samples from different location
- Shear stress: product degradants and Impurities, specifically size variants and sub-visible particulates may be impacted by the mixing process, due to shear and air/protein/mixer and impeller surface interaction during the mixing process while in severe cases, the appearance of the bulk may change (e.g., become more turbid).

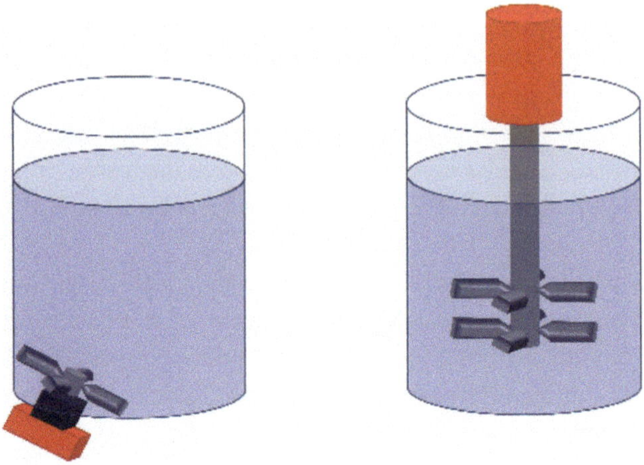

Fig. 2 Top mounted and bottom mounted stirrer.

To achieve the desired product quality and a proper control of the unit operation, the following parameters need to be pre-determined and validated: Mixing Time, Mixing Speed, Product Volume to Mix, Product Temperature.

## 5.6 Filling and aseptic processes

### 5.6.1 Material preparation

When working with sterile products manufactured under aseptic conditions the drug product, containers, and closures are first subjected to washing, siliconization (if needed) and sterilization methods separately, as appropriate, and then brought together (Fig. 3). For example, glass containers are subjected to washing and dry heat; rubber closures are subjected to washing, siliconization and moist heat; and liquid dosage forms are subjected to filtration. Each of these manufacturing processes requires validation and control and because there is no process to sterilize the product in its final container, it is critical that containers be filled and sealed in an extremely high-quality environment.

Not all the process steps for primary packaging components should be executed in line or in the same location, while this is generally the case for vials other components as stoppers and caps may be received by the manufacturing site as ready to use (RSV – ready to used validated).

The washing step is needed to avoid particulate matter from the starting material being introduced in the aseptic process, while the sterilization step assures that each component is sterilized individually before the aseptic assembly.

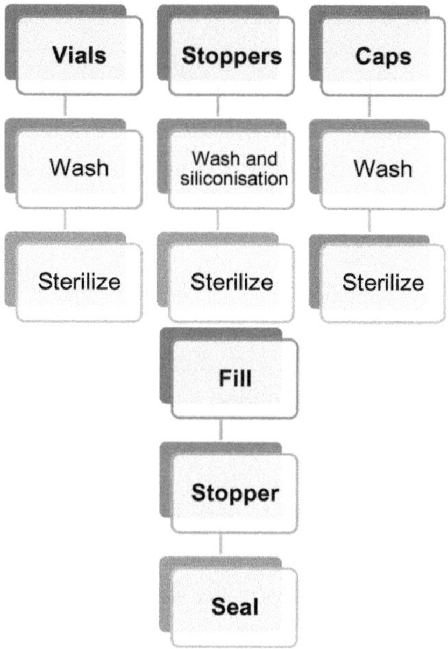


**Fig. 3** Example of material preparation flow.

Indeed, each process could introduce an error that ultimately leads to the distribution of a contaminated product. Any manual or mechanical manipulation of the sterilized drug, components, containers, or closures prior to or during aseptic assembly poses the risk of contamination and thus necessitates careful control.

### *5.6.2 Filling machine technology*

Two different technologies are commonly available for aseptic filling of a sterile product (RABS and Isolator). The advantages and criteria of selection are presented in the following sections.

### *5.6.3 cRABS (restricted access barrier systems)*

RABS provides an enclosed environment that reduces the risk of contaminating the product, containers, closures, and direct contact surfaces. It grants superior protection than conventional cleanroom operations by providing a level of separation between operator and product. Additional details and a full definition of RABS is provided by Lysfjord (2005).

The configurations of RABS include:

- ISO Class 5 (Class A) environment with unidirectional airflow
- Rigid wall enclosure

- Use of glove port/s, half suit/s, to access all areas of the enclosure during filling operations
- Sterilization-In-Place (SIP) is preferred for contact parts (fluid pathways). Other materials coming from the outside environment must undergo autoclaving prior to RABS entry via aseptic transfer ports.

Since the equipment is open to the surrounding room, the background environment should meet grade B.

RABS are further divided into two: open RABS (oRABS) or closed RABS (cRABS).

An oRABS can either have a dedicated air handling system (active) which is completely independent from the room's air supply; or a shared one with the clean-room's downflow (passive), which recycles air from the surrounding environment. Additionally, its barrier doors can be opened for operator intervention at defined risk stages of aseptic processes.

However, cRABS provide a higher level of contamination control since its barrier doors remain closed from the last bio-decontamination through the initial set-up. It also has a dedicated air handling system which will circulate within the barriers. cRABS also makes use of a gaseous decontamination system (Fig. 4).

### 5.6.4 Isolator

An isolator is a completely sealed system with a complete separation of operator and process area. Doors cannot be opened during production, which makes it possible to operate isolators in a class C cleanroom environment.

Isolators are typically equipped with a fully reproducible and validated system for bio-decontamination (mostly H2O2) and a process air handling unit that ensures temperature control by heating or cooling, as well as permanent overpressure control of the process area compared to the operator environment in order to avoid ingress of contaminated air.

Isolators also provide a higher level of protection toward both the operator and the product when handling potent drugs.

The utilization of isolator technology to minimize human interventions in processing areas may result in a significant decrease in the risk of microbiological contamination of aseptically manufactured products from the environment. There are many possible designs of isolators and transfer devices. The isolator and the background environment should be designed so that the required air quality for the respective zones can be realized.

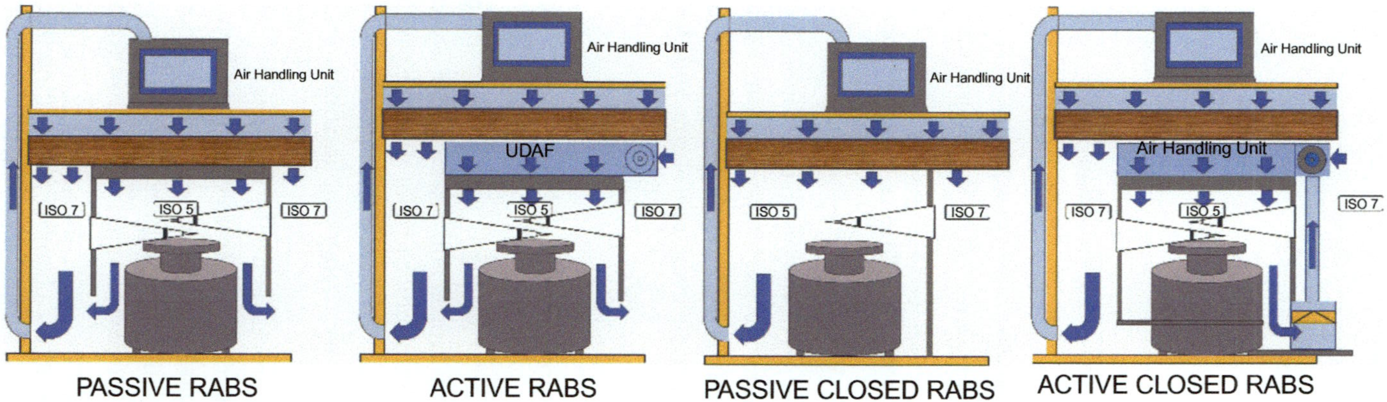


**Fig. 4** Illustrative differences of RABS.

| Isolator | RABS |
|---|---|
| ✔ **Advantages** | |
| • High sterility levels | • Versatility |
| • Reduced volume occupation | • Easily installable in pre-existing facilities |
| • Prolonged operational time | • Possibility of retrofitting |
| • Operator convenience | • Lower capital expenditures |
| • Lower operating expenditures | |
| ✖ **Drawbacks** | |
| • High capital expenditures | • Higher operating costs |
| • Long time required for biodecontamination | • Lower SAL |
| • Effort for H2O2 cycle development and validation | • Not recommended for highly potent |

**Fig. 5** Isolator and RABS comparison (RABS vs. Isolator—Choosing the Right Isolation Technology, 2019).

Isolators are constructed of various materials more or less prone to puncture and leakage. Transfer devices may vary from a single door to double door designs to fully sealed systems incorporating sterilization mechanisms.

For a more detailed comparison of isolators and RABS see Fig. 5.

## 5.7 Lyophilization

Products are manufactured in the lyophilized form due to their instability when in solution.

Lyophilization or freeze drying is a process in which water is removed from a product after it is frozen and placed under a vacuum, allowing the ice to change directly from solid to vapor without passing through a liquid phase. The process consists of three separate, unique, and interdependent processes; freezing, primary drying (sublimation), and secondary drying (desorption).

The lyophilization process generally includes the following steps:

- Transporting the partially stoppered containers from the filling machine to the lyophilizer and loading into the chamber under aseptic conditions.
- Freezing the solution by placing the partially stoppered containers on cooled shelves in a freeze-drying chamber or pre-freezing in another chamber.
- Applying a vacuum to the chamber and heating the shelves in order to evaporate the water from the frozen state.

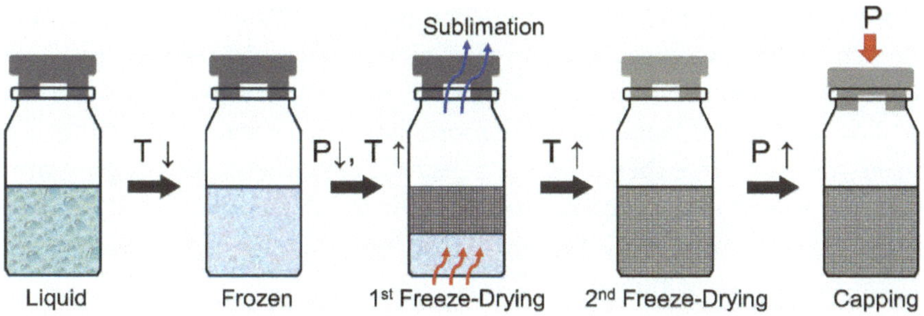


**Fig. 6** Example of lyophilization cycle.

- Complete stoppering of the vials usually by hydraulic or screw rod stoppering mechanisms installed in the lyophilizers (Fig. 6).

Lyophilization is often the most expensive step in Fill-Finish operation of sterile products. This is due to the technical complexity and the length of the process steps that is usually over a few days while filtration and filling are occurring within hours.

Due to the criticality of this step and the line occupation cause by lyophilization, filling lines are often design with more than one equivalent lyophilizator available. This allow to manufacture in parallel multiple batches limiting the time in which the filling machine is on hold waiting the lyophilization step to be completed. Additionally, having more than one equivalent lyo-chamber is a good practice for risk limitation as manufacturing can continue while one of the lyophilizator is under maintenance.

## 5.8 Capping

Capping equipment used in good manufacturing practice (GMP) manufacturing features different designs and a variety of adjustable process parameters. Capping is the last step that assures the packaging container closure.

## 5.9 Visual inspection

USP-1790 Visual Inspection of Injections (2021) clearly establish the expectation that each unit of injectable product needs to be inspected as part of manufacturing process. The intent of this inspection is the detection and removal of any observed defect especially in terms of visible particulate matter and physical defects of the primary packaging configuration.

Manual visual inspection is the most common method for performing 100% visual inspection of parenteral liquids and remains a critical procedure that all manufacturers must continue to perform. Manual Visual Inspection is defined by USP-1790 as the reference inspection method described in all of the major pharmacopeias. It consists of viewing filled and sealed containers under controlled conditions. This process may be aided by the use of a tool to allow consistent examination of more than one container at a time. The quality decision, to either accept or reject the container is made by a trained person. Inspection is a probabilistic process, and detection rates <100% are to be expected, especially for smaller or low-contrast defects (USP-1790 Visual Inspection of Injections, 2021).

Semi-automated visual inspection combines automated material handling of the containers to be inspected with human vision and judgment to make the decision to accept or reject.

Automated visual inspection (AVI) combines automated material handling of the containers with electronic sensing of product appearance. Containers that do not meet pre-programmed acceptance criteria are automatically rejected by the machine. Automated visual inspection, with its higher throughput and lower running costs, provides indeed an effective alternative to manual inspection. Automated visual inspection has improved significantly over the last decade with digitalization and data processing, offering manufacturers a consistent process not subject to fatigue or mood (Flaquiere and Malhete, 2020).

On top of defining the best technology to perform visual inspection, it is primarily important to have a clear definition of the defect to be identified and the correlated criticality.

The manufacturer define, for each product, a dedicated defect list and assigned for each type of defect a specific criticality level (Critical, Major, Minor).

Depending by the associated criticality, the number of defect allowed per batch vary.

For sterile product, defect are usually classified by the primary packaging container in scope and the presence of extraneous matter in the product (Fig. 7).

| Defect on Vial | Defect on Stopper | Defect on Cap | Extraneous Matter | Product Incompliance |
|---|---|---|---|---|
| •Scratch glass<br>•Cracked glass<br>•Glass deformed<br>•Broken container<br>•... | •Missing stopper<br>•Incompliant stopper<br>•Damaged stopper<br>•... | •Dents<br>•Tears<br>•Wrinkles<br>•... | •Particles<br>•Fibers<br>•Hair<br>•Glass<br>•Metal<br>•... | •Empty vial<br>•Underdosed<br>•Overdosed<br>•Missing part (e.g. missing flip-off)<br>•Incompliant product |

**Fig. 7** Example of defect list for visual inspection.

A topic of particular concern is the presence of particles in the product as this may represent a severe risk for patient safety. The presence of particles in an injectable drug product is regulated in the harmonized pharmacopeia chapters USP <788>, Ph.Eur. 2.9.19, and JP 6.07.

During Visual Inspection, personnel and machines are trained and qualified to identify visible particles. During release testing of the product, additional testing for sub-visible particles is conducted.

When particles are identified, a dedicated investigation is required to first identify if the extraneous material is intrinsic, extrinsic to the process or inherent to the product.

- Examples of intrinsic particles are glass and metal where the first may come from the selected primary packaging materials, and the latest from tanks used in manufacturing.
- Example of extrinsic material are fibers and cellulose potentially linked to components used for assembly and packaging
- Inherent particles are instead particles related to the product itself, these particles may be investigated and characterized by the license holder to determine if it can be accepted or production changes are necessary. An example of inherent particles is protein aggregation with silicon oil.

A particle classification is needed to perform a risk evaluation and product quality impact assessment.

# 6. Packaging materials

## 6.1 Introduction and definition

Section 5.6.1 already provided an overview of packaging components that are used for products that are sterile filled. Additional layers of protection are applied to the product by packaging materials guaranteeing a proper product identification and protection.

**Primary packaging** are those that are in direct physical contact with the product.

- vial/syringe
- stopper
- aluminum cap and flip-off

**Secondary packaging** is the exterior packaging of the primary packaging that groups packages and further protects or labels the drug product. Secondary packaging's main purpose is branding display, logistical purposes, and protecting and collating individual units during storage

- label
- leaflet

- folding box

**Tertiary packaging:** facilitates the protection, handling, and transportation of a series of sales units or secondary packages in order to group everything into unit loads during transit. The consumer rarely sees this type of packaging.

- shipping box

## 6.2 General consideration and requirement

When selecting primary packaging materials, interactions between the container and the contents must be investigated.

Product/component stability and compatibility are confirmed during the primary research and development stage. There are numerous possibilities of interactions between primary packaging materials and pharmaceutical products, such as:

- the release of chemicals from components of the packaging materials;
- the release of visible and/or subvisible particles;
- the absorption or adsorption of pharmaceutical components by the packaging materials;
- chemical reactions between the pharmaceutical product and the packaging materials;
- the degradation of packaging components in contact with the pharmaceutical products;
- the influence of the manufacturing process (e.g., sterilization) on the container.

The active pharmaceutical ingredients should remain within their specification limits over the shelf life of the pharmaceutical product. The question of whether a packaging will provide the required protection for the pharmaceutical product and the required stability over a certain time period can only be answered by means of real-time stability studies. Such studies must evaluate the changes in the quality of the product, in contact with its packaging, during a period equivalent to its intended shelf life.

In addition, packaging materials (primary/secondary/tertiary) must meet the following requirements:

- it must preserve the physical properties of all dosage forms and protect them against damage or breakage;
- it must not alter the identity of the product;
- it must preserve the characteristic properties of the product, so that the latter complies with its specifications;

- it must protect the product against undesirable or adulterating chemical, biological or physical entities.

## 6.3 Packaging material incoming control

Microbiological contamination of starting materials should be minimal. Specification documents should include requirements for microbiological quality when the need for this has been indicated by monitoring.

Additionally to packaging components mentioned in the previous chapter, when handling sterile product before final container closure, containers and materials liable to generate fibers should be minimized in clean areas.

## 6.4 Primary packaging material preparation

Available sterilization methods:
- Sterilization by heat (e.g., depyrogenation tunnel)
- Moist heat (e.g., autoclave for stoppers and cap)
- Additional sterilization method as sterilization by radiation/ethylene oxide

All sterilization processes should be validated and the validity of the process should be verified at scheduled intervals, at least annually, and whenever significant modifications have been made to the equipment.

The interval between the washing and drying and the sterilization of components, containers and equipment as well as between their sterilization and use should be minimized and subject to a time-limit appropriate to the storage conditions.

## 6.5 Container closure for primary packaging material

Closures, as primary packaging components, are of critical importance and must be carefully selected. They are an essential component of the container and, as such, an integral part of the drug preparation. A container type, which does not require a removable closure at the time of administration, is usually preferred since such a container/closure system avoids, or at least minimizes, the risk of biological and other contamination as well as tampering.

For parenteral preparations, the combination of glass containers and elastomeric closures, usually secured by an aluminum cap, is widely used. Typical examples are infusion bottles, injection vials and prefilled syringes. The rubber closures used within such a system must be selected in accordance with the intended purpose. Most often, improper rubber closures are the cause of incompatibility between the packaging and the drug. A special design of stopper may also be required for some pharmaceutical production processes such as lyophilization.

Containers should be closed by appropriately validated methods. The container closure system for aseptically filled vials is not fully integral until the aluminum cap has been crimped into place on the stoppered vial. Crimping of the cap should therefore be performed as soon as possible after stopper insertion.

## 6.6 Secondary packaging material

A secondary packaging component means a packaging component that is not and will not be in direct contact with the dosage form.

Secondary packaging consists of:

- Labels, inks and adhesive materials (e.g., glue);
- Package inserts for patients;
- Blister/carton

Secondary packaging material components in clinical phase and commercial phase may be extremely different. From a regulatory standpoint, manufacturing and packaging of all pharmaceutical products must comply with cGMP requirements, regardless of clinical or commercial applications but this can be achieve implementing different processes.

For example, the double-blinding of clinical packs requires using more barcode labeling and database management on the line.

Clinical runs tend to be short, with extensive documentation and audit trail requirements, so line set-ups can be long.

Commercial packaging is a longer run with bigger batch size and requires investment in automated quality control, such as scanners for visual inspection.

## 6.7 Tertiary packaging material

Any business that ships goods uses tertiary packaging in the distribution process. Tertiary packaging is there to protect both the product and the packaging that sits underneath when being transported from one destination to another

Each single component of the packaging systems needs to be qualified and should be able to sustain stresses that are typical to pharmaceutical distribution (Worldwide by road, by plane, oversee). Pre-defined stress condition defined by ASTM standard are applied during configuration development and material qualification.

## 6.8 Equipment overview

The packaging operations of sterile pharma form is a highly automated process involving mainly mechanical operations, biocompatibility considerations are still involved in material selection especially when dealing with mechanical device. The main difference between packaging equipment for pharma and other commercial fields is the number and accuracy of quality controlled applied to the goods.

For standard configuration, three type of equipment are installed on shop floor:

- Labeling machine: product identification, label printing and application on primary packaging container
- Cartoning machine: product identification, packaging of the labelled primary container in the secondary box, leaflet insertion, printing of variable data and (optional) addition of components for product administration in the box as needles.

These machines are usually named by the concept of top loading or side loading depending on the direction in which the primary packaging container and leaflet are inserted in the folding box. In addition to the direction of insertion of the primary packaging container, another important feature that will affect the mechanism of function of case packer machine is the presence of folding box partition and plastic trays for package configuration including more than one container

- Case packer: Arrangement of secondary box in the shipping container, product counting and reconciliation, data management.

## 6.9 Medical device and combination product

Medical device and combination product is an area that is rapidly growing in relevance when dealing with pharmaceutical product. Medical device are indeed supporting patient's experience and safety during product administration.

In this chapter, only a brief definition of medical device and combination product is provided as the field is wide and a dedicated full chapter will be required:

- **Medical device**: An instrument, apparatus, implement, machine, implant which does not achieve its primary intended purposes through chemical action within or on the body of man or other animals and which is not dependent upon being metabolized for the achievement of its primary intended purposes.

- **Combination product**: Therapeutic and diagnostic products that combine drugs, devices, and/or biological products (FDA)
    - o product vial and auto-injector
    - o Pre-filled Syringes (PFS)

## 7. Cold chain

Little different type of cold chain packaging systems are available, they are grouped as active, passive and hybrid, where:

- Active systems: Active thermal systems do not use any phase change materials (PCM) such as water/ice or dry ice. These systems use mechanical or electric systems powered by an energy source, combined by thermostatic control to maintain proper product temperatures.
- Passive systems: Passive thermal systems commonly use phase change materials (PCM) such as water/ice or dry ice. These shipping systems are the most basic and cost effective.

The most suitable cold chain system is selected based on the quantity of the goods to be shipped, the complexity of the supply chain and the temperature requirement to be granted:

Active thermal systems provide:

- Highest cost
- Highest temperature accuracy
- High reliability
- Standard/off the shelf sizes only—no custom sizes feasible
- Easy to use

Passive thermal systems provide:

- Lowest cost
- Lowest temperature accuracy
- High reliability with proper procedures
- Standard/off the shelf and custom sizes may not require tooling
- Phase Change Material conditioning required—hardest to use

## 8. Future trends

Pharmaceutical manufacturing of sterile products is rapidly evolving with the availability of new molecules targeting different patient populations. Recently, great emphasis is given to the possibility of cure of rare diseases or to treat well-known diseases with different technology such as Cell & Gene therapies (CG&T). While this is bringing hope to patients, it comes with new challenges for Pharmaceutical plants designed to produce a high quantity of blockbuster products.

Pharmaceutical companies that are active in this field need to deal with challenges as

- Super small batch size and complexity in manufacturing (e.g., quick change over, equipment design, production on demand and knowledge management, personalized medicine and patient centricity)
  - o Increased focus on equipment able to manufacture small batch size reducing product losses (e.g., modular solution for filling and robotic solution for secondary packaging)
- CG&T
  - o Quick turnaround (from patient to same patient in one day)
  - o Limited temperature and product stability (extreme cold chain condition)

Not only the treatment opportunities are evolving, patient centricity is becoming the primary focus and a game changer in market access strategies. Opportunity to administer treatment in a more conformable set up as home administration, or self-administration that will reduce hospitalization time and improve patient quality of life are emerging trends in the pharmaceutical space. This translates in an increasing need to have medical devices and automated components to facilitate the administration of the product. While the goal is clear, the possibility and the expertise required, that combines mechanical, biochemical and automation, are evolving and getting closer to each other re-designing modern facilities.

High levels of automation and paper-less plants are already a reality in many pharmaceutical plants, this evolution was not only pushed over the years from the clear benefit that automation can bring to complex operation but even from increasing health authorities' requirement in terms of product safety and traceability.

Implementation of serialization and single unit code are only a couple of recent examples on how regulatory agencies are stressing the need to have full control on medicine distribution to confirm quality.

## Glossary

**Drug substance** Drug substance is an active ingredient that is intended to furnish pharmacological activity or other direct effect in the diagnosis, cure, mitigation, treatment, or prevention of disease or to affect the structure or any function of the human body, but does not include intermediates used in the synthesis of such ingredient.

**Drug product** The finished dosage form that contains a drug substance, generally, but not necessarily in association with other active or inactive ingredients.

**Bioburden** The total number of microorganisms associated with a specific item prior to sterilization.

**Endotoxin** A pyrogenic product (e.g., lipopolysaccharide) present in the bacterial cell wall. Endotoxin can lead to reactions in patients receiving injections ranging from fever to death.

**Sterilizing grade filter** A filter that, when challenged with the Bacterium Brevundimonas diminuta at the minimum concentration of $10^7$ colony forming units (CFU) per $cm^2$ of filter surface area, will produce a sterile effluent (ASTM F838).

**Terminal sterilization** Terminal sterilization usually involves filling and sealing product containers under high-quality environmental conditions. Products are filled and sealed in this type of environment to minimize the microbial and particulate content of the in-process product and to help ensure that the subsequent sterilization process is successful. In most cases, the product, container, and closure have low bioburden, but they are not sterile. The product in its final container is then subjected to a sterilization process such as heat or irradiation.

**Particulate matter** Mobile undissolved particles, other than gas bubbles, unintentionally present in the solutions (USP 788—Particulate Matter in Injections, 2012).

**Visible particles** Approximately 100–150 μm and larger, which can be spotted with the naked eye during visual inspection and without any outside assistance such as magnifying glasses or microscopes.

**Sub-visible particles** Approximately 0.1–100 μm. Sub-visible particles are usually defined as being in the size range 0.1–100 μm, often above the upper size limit for measurement by size-exclusion chromatography but not sufficiently large to be detectable by eye.

## References


Annex 1—Manufacture of Sterile Medicinal Products: *EudraLex*, vol. 4, Brussels, 2008, November 25, EU guidelines to good manufacturing practice medicinal products for human and veterinary use.

FDA: Guidance for industry, In *Container closure systems for packaging human drugs and biologics*, 1999, May, U.S. Department of Health and Human Services, Food and Drug Administration, Center for Drug Evaluation and Research (CDER), Center for Biologics Evaluation and Research (CBER).

FDA: Guidance for industry, In Q7 *Good manufacturing, practice guidance for active pharmaceutical ingredients*, 2016, September, U.S. Department of Health and Human Services, Food and Drug Administration, Center for Drug Evaluation and Research (CDER), Center for Biologics Evaluation and Research (CBER).

FDA. (n.d.). Sterile drug products produced by aseptic processing—current good manufacturing practices, U.S. Department of Health and Human Services, Food and Drug Administration, Center for Drug Evaluation and Research (CDER), Center for Biologics Evaluation and Research (CBER), Office of Regulatory Affairs (ORA).

Flaquiere A, Malhete J: *Qualification of manual visual inspection still critical*, 2020, March 19, Retrieved from pda.org https://www.pda.org/pda-letter-portal/home/full-article/qualification-of-manual-visual-inspection-still-critical.

Global Regulatory Authority Websites. (n.d.). Retrieved from pda.org https://www.pda.org/scientific-and-regulatory-affairs/regulatory-resources/global-regulatory-authority-websites.

Lysfjord J: ISPE definition: restricted access barrier system (RABS) for aseptic processing, *Official Mag ISPE* 25(6):1–3, 2005.
RABS vs. Isolator—Choosing the Right Isolation Technology. (2019, August 23). Retrieved from pharmablog.syntegon.com: https://pharmablog.syntegon.com/2019/08/23/rabs-vs-isolator-choosing-the-right-isolation-technology/.
Kimberly Steffen and Sal M. Giglia, (n.d.). Maximizing the performance and efficiency of your sterilizing-grade filtration. Bioprocess Online.
The European Regulatory System, A consistent approach to medicines regulation. (2016). Retrieved from ema.europa.eu: https://www.ema.europa.eu/en/documents/leaflet/european-regulatory-system-medicines-european-medicines-agency-consistent-approach-medicines_en.pdf.
USP 788—Particulate Matter in Injections: *USP 788—particulate matter in injections*, 2012, July 1, The United States Pharmacopeial Convention.
USP-1790 Visual Inspection of Injections: *USP-1790 visual inspection of injections*, 2021, May 1.

## Further reading

Chakradhar Padala FJ: Impact of uncontrolled vs controlled rate freeze-thaw technologies on process performance and product quality, *PDA J Pharm Sci Technol*, 2010, July.
European Commission—Enterprise And Industry Directorate-General: EU GMP Annex 1: manufacture of sterile medicinal product, In *EudraLex—the rules governing medicinal products in the European Union*, vol. 4, Brussels, 2008, November 25, EU Guidelines to Good Manufacturing Practice Medicinal Products for Human and Veterinary Use.
Hammer C: *Carton packaging systems for parenterals. ONdrugDelivery Magazine, Issue 71*, Oct 2016, pp 76–78.
Restricted Access Barrier System (RABS) Retrofits for Existing Equipment. (2015, June 3). Retrieved from pharmablog.syntego: https://pharmablog.syntegon.com/2015/06/03/rabs-2/.
The Lyophilization Basics. (2020, March 19) Retrieved from Lyophilizationworld: https://www.lyophilizationworld.com/post/2020/03/19/the-lyophilization-process.
World Health Organization: *Annex 6—WHO good manufacturing practices for sterile pharmaceutical products*, vol. 961, 2011, WHO Technical Report.

# Index

Note: Page numbers followed by "*f*" indicate figures and "*t*" indicate tables.

## D



## E



## F

## W



## Z

FSC
www.fsc.org
MIX
Papier | Fördert
gute Waldnutzung
FSC® C083411

Kolibri 360 GmbH
Ferdinand-Jühlke-Straße 7
99095 Erfurt, Deutschland
produktsicherheit@kolibri360.de